My Knee Replacement Adventure:

Getting Back the Bend

by
Hertha James

Powerword Publications
Muddy Horse Coaching
hertha.james@xtra.co.nz
www.herthamuddyhorse.com

Disclaimer of Liability
This book describes my personal experiences and some of the exercises I found helpful. It in no way purports to tell a full story about knee replacements generally or suggest that professional physical therapy may not be useful for many people. Since people are all different in age, gender, health, lifestyle, and fitness levels, my experiences are personal. But they will hopefully give those contemplating new knees an idea of what to expect.

Risk Radar: it's important to look after brand-new knees by avoiding twisting, jolting, stumbling and falling. It pays to err on the side of slow and safe.

James, Hertha. *My Knee Replacement Adventure: Getting Back the Bend*

Cover photo: My horse, Boots, helping me with my knee-bending exercises.

Illustrations:
Some illustrations are taken from video footage, so sharpness was sacrificed to capture specific moments.

Table of Contents

Chapter 1: The Decision

When it was painful to walk to my front gate, it was clear that I would have to become proactive about seeing to my knees. I was 69. My husband had his own health challenges. We want to continue to live independently in our rural home for as long as possible.

Six months earlier, when the knees had started to seriously affect walking out and about for pleasure, my general practitioner had suggested x-rays to give us a basis of comparison in the future. Knee replacements are done in the public health system, but to even qualify for the waiting list, it seems a person has to be pretty much immobilised according to an official checklist.

Since I was (slowly and painfully) doing all my horse chores and playing with my horse each morning for 1-2 hours and still able to drive short distances comfortably, I was well short of getting on such a list without recourse to dishonesty.

Stem Cell Treatment?

For a while I dabbled with the idea of stem cell injections derived from factors in my own blood. However, the science is hazy about how this might grow new cartilage where cartilage was totally missing from half of each knee.

The people in my area offering such a stem cell procedure were only able to say that 80% of their patients reported a positive effect. Privacy rules made it impossible to speak to their clients. This was not enough information to make me confident about giving stem cells a try.

Recently a study has been set up in Australia to do clinical trials testing the stem cell procedure on knees devoid of cartilage. In another ten or twenty years it may be an option. Since there are many reasons for knee problems, stem cell therapy may well work for some of the conditions.

Medication

Pain relief medication is the first option offered for chronic knee discomfort. However, I'm well aware that pain medications all have an adverse effect on the kidneys (and gut and who knows what other body parts). Occasionally, to help sleep at night, I used dissolvable aspirin to take the edge off the pain.

I had already had an unhappy experience with acetaminophen which has brand names Paracetamol or Tylenol. A sore elbow caused me to take Paracetamol in 6-hourly doses for several days in a row. The result was not pretty. I developed a swelling in my neck and a rash.

My doctor suggested I pay for an immediate ultrasound to ensure the lump wasn't cancerous. The doctor at the ultrasound clinic said it did not look problematic and to give it three months. He described it as an inflammation of lymph nodes which can be caused by a variety of things.

The clinic which houses my doctor has a sign that says, "Let us know right away if you have a rash". It usually takes several days to get an appointment, so I took my rash in without an appointment. I told them about my rash at reception, but no attention was given to it and after waiting for five hours to be seen by the on-call doctor, I took my rash home. It gradually faded over several weeks.

Meanwhile, my doctor had organized a public health system specialist to see my lump. When the appointment rolled around about three weeks later, my lump was just a memory, but I went along in the hope of seeing if this specialist might be able to link the lump (and rash) to the Paracetamol.

Three hours after my appointment time, after 6 p.m., I was finally seen by the specialist's apprentice. He was perturbed about not finding a lump. I explained how it had gradually reduced and tried to explain my concern with the drugs which may have caused the (now phantom) lump. He called the specialist who was even more annoyed at not finding the promised lump. He also had absolutely no interest in my queries about the lump/rash/Paracetamol connection. Instead, he booked me for a biopsy into a non-existing lump............... a sign of overwork?

At this point, I realised that a specialist is probably no longer at his best after the dinner hour and took myself home. The biopsy appointment duly arrived. I cancelled it and wrote the specialist a letter of explanation.

Other than taking the Paracetamol for my aching elbow so I could sleep, nothing else had changed, so I am now wary of taking more than one occasional dose of Paracetamol. When I Googled the side effects of this drug, I came upon posts by hordes of people who experienced all kinds of negative side effects from it.

I had taken glucosamine and chondroitin for many years. Then I switched to Arthrem for a couple of years. It seems that Arthrem also affects kidney function.

While researching and thinking about what to do, I came across a paper from an international group of orthopaedic specialists and rheumatologists. The paper looked in detail at the benefit/harm caused by the various medications and 'helping aids' used around the world. It was an eye opener. Quite often the difference between benefit and harm was worryingly small. The only item with no harmful side effect was using a cane!

Below is the link to a Osteoarthritis Research Society International (OARSI) PDF document compiled in 2013, if you want to have a closer look at the variety of medications which are prescribed for knee pain. https://www.oarsi.org/sites/default/files/docs/2014/non surgical treatment of knee oa march 2014.pdf. (Accessed November 2, 2018.)

Surgery It Is

Having so far managed to live without regular prescribed medication, I was not keen to begin relying on pain killers, with their negative effect on my kidneys and digestive system. The only choice that remained was surgical intervention.

I asked my doctor to organize a private consultation with an orthopaedic surgeon. Going private was the only way to have new knees in a timely manner, before things deteriorated even further. The stronger the muscles are before surgery, the easier the recuperation.

On entering the surgeon's office, an x-ray of my knees, taken six months earlier, was already on his huge screen. It was a jolt to see such a clear picture of my inner knees totally devoid of cartilage. Plus, there was six months of wear and tear on top of what the x-ray showed.

The surgeon agreed with my prognosis. I could either pop pills until the cows come home or have knee replacements. Since my discomfort walking and sitting at my computer for any length of time was increasing rapidly, it was time to decide.

When the surgeon ascertained that I was generally healthy, not on any regular medications and as active as my knees allowed, he suggested that I have both knees done at the same time.

This appealed to me because if only one was done, the sorry state of the unoperated knee would not help much in the recovery of the operated knee. It also meant only one episode of anaesthetics and post-op narcotics, plus one recovery period. Since I was paying for the procedure and hospital stay, it also made sense in terms of expense.

Chapter 2: The Decline

The highlights of my sports career occurred between ages 13 and 18. I remember daily running the perimeter of the school sports field to add to the school total to run across Canada from the Pacific to the Atlantic (4,444 kilometres or 2,761 miles).

I was keen on athletics and played softball, basketball and volleyball throughout high school. My summer job was in the Calgary Children's Zoo, as animal keeper and host to the visitors.

After three years at university, I moved to New Zealand to work in Wellington Zoo. Then I spent several years back in Canada working as animal keeper and handler on a film set in the Rocky Mountains. This was a challenge during both winter and summer. I also pursued my main passion of keeping and riding horses.

I did a year of teacher-training in New Zealand, followed by 23 years of teaching science and biology. Plus, time daily with my horses. A fair amount of energy is required to look after horses and still have time to ride on top of a full-time job and a family.

Eventually I exchanged teaching for part-time work as a high school librarian. Working part time gave me a few extra hours each morning to ride and explore equine clicker training.

Aged 61, I found it harder and harder to ride my wide-beamed quarter horse. X-rays showed that my hips were developing bone spurs. So I gave up riding and began Horse Agility, which is done on the ground with the horse. We had fun learning to navigate a monthly series of obstacles to take part in a low-key international video clip competition.

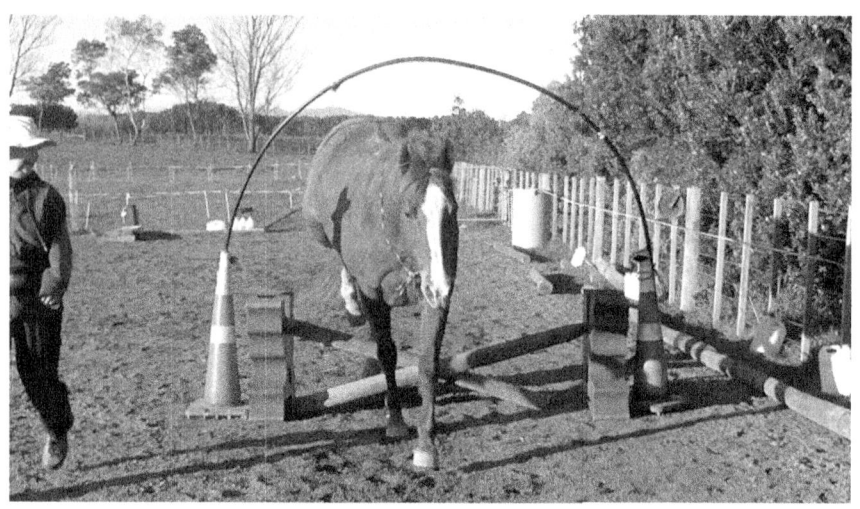

A Horse Agility obstacle with my horse, Boots. This was back in the day when I could still jog

A year before my 69th birthday, jogging became problematic, so Boots and I were restricted to entering the 'walk only' classes. All my life I had walked my dogs and horses several kilometres a day.

Gradually it became more and more painful to walk to the nearby river with my horse. Eventually I had to give up walking and ride my bike with Boots walking or trotting alongside.

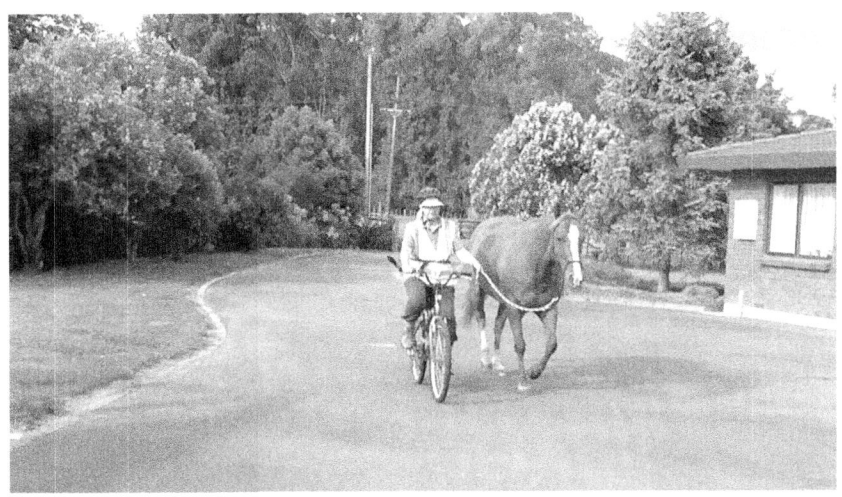

When walking became too painful, the only way to take Boots out for jaunts was by riding my bike.

Walking continued to become more and more painful (both knees equally sore) until any time I wanted to go further than the front gate for fresh air, I had to ride my bicycle. Even getting around the supermarket became an effort.

NOTES:

NOTES:

Chapter 3: The Surgery

The surgeon explained that each replacement takes about an hour. If my vital signs showed stress after the first operation, the second one could be postponed.

It was only a three-week wait between making the decision to go ahead with the knee replacements, and having them done.

During those weeks we were immersed in the adventure (trauma) of having a new kitchen fitted, so I did not dwell a lot on the upcoming operation. Neither did I have time to research the details about the total knee replacement process and the challenges inherent in the recovery. Possibly this was a good thing.

I was asked to stop taking any medication or supplements for two weeks before the surgery. This included the multivitamin taken to maintain my vitamin B12 level. All these substances can interfere with the anaesthetic during the operation.

The Scary Nurse

The private hospital in our little city is new and welcoming. Once payment was made, the care was excellent. I'd been there before when my husband underwent procedure.

Prior to my pre-operation appointment with the enrolment nurse, the hospital sent out several pages of questions requiring details of my medical history, allergies, sensitivities, and so on. During the appointment, the enrolment nurse entered all the particulars from the questionnaire into the hospital computer program and clarified any points.

The other part of the enrolment nurse's job was to describe the recovery procedure in some detail. Her information, she said, was gleaned from what patients have told her.

She made sure I realized that I was about to have major surgery. She outlined the risk factors. She emphasized the nature, duration and pain of the recovery process. She wanted to be sure about my determination to go ahead. She gave me a lot to think about, but I felt like I was in an extremely narrow space with 'forward' as the only way out.

The Day Arrives

My operation was in the morning, meaning a 7:30 a.m. arrival at the hospital. Nil by mouth after midnight. I packed my bag and hoped for the best.

I was taken to the private room that would be mine for the seven-day stay. Almost immediately the surgeon and anaesthetist arrived for a quick chat. Things all happened rapidly. In no time I was in a hospital gown and being wheeled to the operating theatre where the surgeon was finishing off his pep talk (or was it a 'prep talk') to his team.

When the surgeon asked how I was feeling, I replied that I hoped he was a morning person.

I'd never had an epidural before, so I focused on my five breaths in and five breaths out. It was all very efficient and painless. A nurse engaged me in conversation while I sat on the edge of a gurney and the surgeon behind me said he found a perfect spot to insert the needle and that was pretty much it until I was in the recovery room after the operations.

Evidently the epidural numbs the entire lower body. Then the other anaesthetics are added. When I later read through the itemized list of things I had paid for, seeing the saw blades made me happy about this precaution.

Both knees were done. The surgeon was happy with how it went.

Hospital Time

For the first day and a half, a catheter collected my urine, so I could stay in bed. When the protective bandage was removed, the wounds showed up beautifully stitched and protected with a transparent water-proof dressing.

Right from the start, the nurses quizzed me about sensation in my toes and suggested ankle movement and thigh contractions to the best of my ability. All movement helps prevent blood clots.

I was hooked to an IV for antibiotics and a patient-controlled morphine pump. This is set up so pressing a button delivers morphine with a minimum of ten-minute intervals. It gave me the comforting feeling of having a little bit of control.

Usually the IV drip also contains a secondary back-up of Paracetamol to help control pain, but due to my past negative response to this, it was omitted. My blood oxygen occasionally dropped a bit lower than it should, so I was asked to breathe deeply every time my vital signs were checked, and I had oxygen nibs in my nose.

The surgeon kept a close watch and debated whether I needed a blood transfusion due to low oxygen levels, but eventually decided I was okay without it. The surgeon visited every day without fail, even on Sunday. He checked the wounds and we had a chat about how things were progressing. The main post-surgery problems are blood clots and infection. An infection anywhere in the body can travel to the knee surgery site.

The nurses were kind and helpful. I was lucky to have a student nurse in the mix, so an extra person to cheer-lead me to new heights of endeavour. It is interesting to note the effect the nurses' attitudes had on the way I responded to their suggestions.

Most of the nurses used positive reinforcement. In other words, they commented on my positive achievements and gave helpful suggestions on what I could try next. One nurse, however, thought she was helpful by being stern when I didn't feel up to sitting in a chair for a meal, do enough moving of my knees by rubbing a plastic bag along the floor, or if I turned down the intensity of the continuous passive movement machine when the pain became excruciating in my left knee.

One of my key interests is exploring positive reinforcement in the context of training horses. Rewarding positive achievements and making gentle suggestions results in a horse keen to repeat the things that earn the reward.

It is interesting to note how the different attitudes of the nurses affected my willingness to do specific physical therapy. Quite unconsciously, I developed an internal resistance to doing what the stern nurse wanted. In fact, my thoughts turned to outwitting her. I was relieved when she had her days off.

It wasn't until I was home again with lots of time for thinking, that I realized what had happened with the different nursing styles. Being so helpless and vulnerable had obviously returned me to the most basic of emotional responses.

I was lucky that most of the nurses celebrated my smallest achievements and seemed to know exactly when to suggest trying something more. To go home, I had to walk with crutches for a certain distance, use the toilet independently, have had a bowel movement and be able to cope with steps.

On the second day, the catheter and IV were removed. I took antibiotic capsules instead. It was a big moment when I first put my feet on the floor with the help of the nurses, and had the crutches adjusted to the right height.

I gradually learned how to lower myself onto the toilet and put the crutches into a position for easy retrieval, where they wouldn't fall down out of reach. At first the nurses helped directly, but gradually they let me be more and more independent. By midweek I could swing my feet off the bed to the floor on my own and meander to the loo. I only needed help to lift my legs back onto the bed.

At this point, I was introduced to a shiny slippery piece of material that made it easier to scoot my bottom along the bed and move my legs off or onto the bed. I learned how to fold back the blankets before exiting the bed, so I could independently settle back into bed and draw them over me again.

I had an assisted shower midweek. By the end of the week I was able to shower alone. In between showers it was no problem to have a wash and brush my teeth, as I could brace myself against the sink.

The back of my right foot developed what felt like a 'bed sore'. A nurse folded a soft fluffy cloth in half and put it under my ankles, which eased the pressure on the sore spot and made me more comfortable. One of the hardest parts of the early recovery weeks is being restricted to lying on one's back.

Sleep was fairly elusive. I had my radio brought in, which helped pass the nights. The TV in my room helped while away some of the day and I soon had favorite programs to watch. As the week progressed, the night nurse visits became less frequent. I had a lovely night nurse. I also had control of the room's heat pump, so could keep the room at a temperature comfortable for me.

By day six I was able to sit on the edge of the bed and draw both legs up onto the bed together by myself. Each day, more walking and general activity started to show results.

Bowel movements were tricky. For the first three days I had no appetite and ate very little. This was a shame because the food was excellent. By day five the doctor ordered a low-key enema which had a modest effect. Next day brought a heavier-duty enema, which had the desired result.

On day two, I was introduced to the continuous passive motion (CPM) machine. The leg was placed on the machine and it forces the knee to bend and straighten. The angle of the bend can be varied. This was done for one hour on each knee. My right knee coped admirably, the left one not so much. I quickly learned how to control the degree of bend. Some nurses were better than others at getting my leg onto the machine at a comfortable angle.

I convinced the nurses to let me start the motion gently and I would increase it every ten minutes or so. From training horses to be supple, I knew enough about the importance of a warm-up and a cool-down when it comes to muscles. I imagine even traumatised muscles appreciate this.

By day three I was on the machine for two hours morning and another two hours in the late afternoon (an hour for each leg each time). The left knee became quite convinced that it was a torture device.

Evidently some of the knee orthopaedics community no longer believe in the use of these machines. I suppose if it does nothing else, it keeps things moving and helps waylay blood clots.

The whole hospital stay was helped by frequent visits from family and friends. My last hurdle before going home was to prove that I could negotiate a set of steps.

Summary of Achievements for Week One

The time specified is counted in days/weeks after my operation. My operation was at 8 a.m. in the morning, so I'm counting that day as Day 1.

Sleep was elusive and for three or four days I had little appetite.

Day 1

- Remained in bed with morphine pump and catheter, so needed no trips to the loo.

Day 2

- Catheter removed mid-morning.
- Introduced to my crutches.
- Helped to the toilet by nurses.
- Needed help swinging my legs to the floor and back onto the bed again.

- Introduced to the Continuous Passive Motion (CPM) machine for half an hour on each knee. This was increased to an hour for each knee for the next five days in hospital. Right knee coped well; left knee was not so keen.

Day 3

- I could swing my legs (together) off the bed and stand with my crutches.
- Nurses helped me to the bathroom but let me do as much as I could by myself.
- Needed help to lift my legs back up onto the bed.
- Nurses helped me with a short walk in the corridor (with crutches).

Day 4

- Introduced to a piece of slippery material which I put under my butt to help me slide along the bed to get up and slide back in.
- Encouraged to sit in a chair for a meal and to slide my feet back and forth under the chair on a plastic bag. Very painful but I tried.
- Nurse-assisted shower.
- Nurse-accompanied walk in the corridor.
- Night nurse checked up less frequently.

Day 5

- First bowel movement with assistance of an enema.
- Sat in a chair for one or two meals and for doing the 'foot on plastic bag shuffle'. Painful.
- Able to go to bathroom on my own.
- Lifted my legs back onto the bed without help.
- Walked a bit further in the corridor without nurse in attendance.

Day 6

- Showered without supervision. Walked further in corridor.

Day 7

- All the above achievements plus a successful session learning to navigate steps.

NOTES:

Chapter 4: Coming Home and Week 2

Day seven after the operation, I was ready to go home. The requirements were:

- Walk independently with crutches, tick.
- Sit in a chair at a table (painfully), tick.
- Get into and out of bed independently, tick.
- Bowel movement, tick.
- Navigate stairs, tick.

My husband and son had organized:

- A raised toilet seat (hired).
- A firm chair with arms (hired, as we only had soft-seat recliners and dining chairs with no arms).
- A table with wheels (hired, but I later purchased one).
- Large packet of baby wipes.
- Packet of incontinence undies (I only used a few of these but it was a comfort to know I had them).
- A super-long shoe horn (a sock puller-upper would also be useful).
- A long-handled grabbing device to pick things up (hand-me-down from a relative no longer with us).
- A couch moved into the family room, so I could stretch out with my legs up and watch TV.

Other suggestions are:

- Avoid 'slip on' footwear.
- Take up any loose mats from the floor.
- Have simple, easy meals already organized, e.g. soups and frozen meals.
- Have plenty of fruit to snack on.

- Have heating in the bedroom if necessary, because heavy blankets will be impossible. Most houses in New Zealand don't have central heating, so our bedrooms are mostly unheated. In the winter it can be zero degrees Celsius during a frosty night, so I used a space heater until spring rolled around.

My bed and toilet at home were fortunately the same height as those in the hospital. For the toilet I only needed the side of the commode apparatus to lean on to get up and down. The toilet-roll holder fixed into the wall on the other side was robust enough for me to lean on getting up and down.

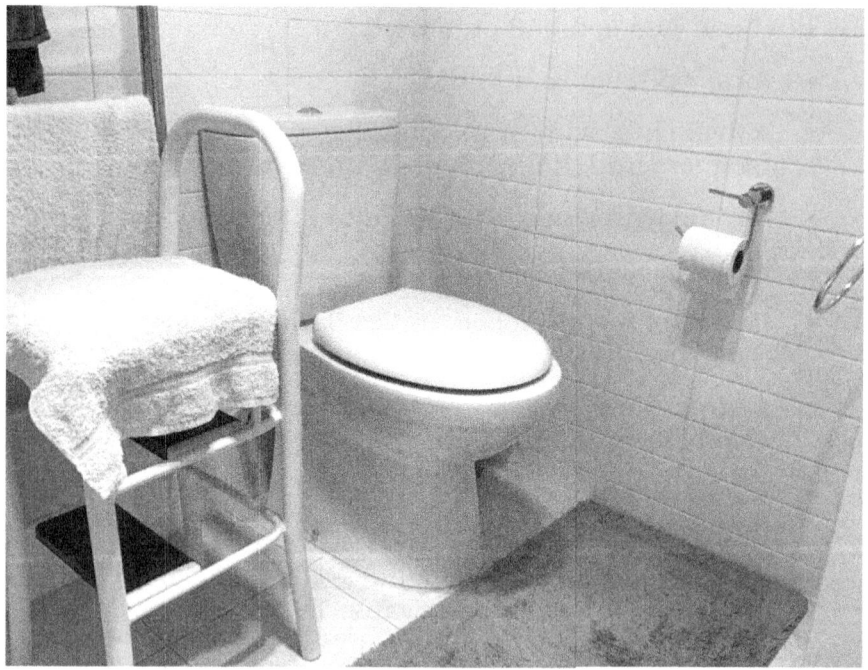

I was soon able to return the rented commode and use the side of this step-stool and the toilet-holder knob to use the toilet safely.

Our car, luckily, was an SUV, so with some excruciating leg-bending, we managed to shoe-horn me in. The nurses came along to help and say good-bye. We stopped at a chemist (drug store) for pain relief (Codeine, Arcoxia) and Aspirin to fend off blood clots. The car ride was distinctly uncomfortable, even with pillows to tuck under my knees to help keep my legs relatively straight.

The main entry to our house has one unusually tall step into the main house. I soon worked out that by using a different door, I could enter and exit using two smaller steps. I had the door frame to brace against for one step, and the wall of the house to lean on at the second smaller step.

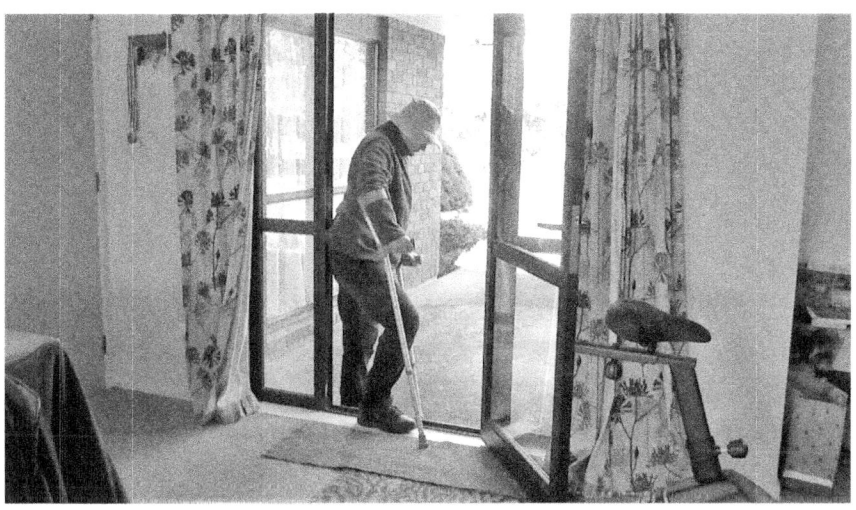

This door has the smallest step to get outside. By bracing my backside against the door frame, and relying on my crutches, I was able to step down sideways.

For the first two days I needed help putting on my socks and trousers, but I soon worked out how to reach down and pull them on. My husband is super-supportive, but it was my job to do everything I could to regain independence. Everything just took a long time to accomplish.

My daytime resting area was a couch in the family room where I could watch TV to help while away the time. The couch is quite low, so to get up I used the wooden end of the couch and a chair on my other side to push myself up. I placed my crutches where they were handy but not about to trip anyone up. The house is all one level, which made moving around straightforward.

I made a conscious decision not to visit my horse, Boots, until I felt a bit more secure. I spent the days alternately sitting, walking and lying down, retiring to bed by 9 p.m. Sleep was difficult because I had never normally slept on my back. Listening to the radio helped, as did listening to audio books which I borrowed from the library.

I was sent home with three medications. Codeine to take 6-hourly as needed for pain, Arcoxia which is for inflammation and pain (one a day) and Aspirin once daily to help avoid blood clots. I tried hard to not take Codeine more than eight-hourly, because it is a major cause of constipation and a very dry mouth.

Details about Week Two After the New Knees

I gradually settled into a routine. Bryan, my very supportive husband, brought me a cup of green tea in bed at 7 a.m.

I walked around the house with my crutches and sat at a table, both of which were painful. I didn't quite trust my stability carrying things in the kitchen, so Bryan made my porridge.

Basically, bouts of sitting and walking were interspersed with reclining on the couch and watching TV or staring happily into space. I had especially stocked up on library books, but my mind was still so fuzzy that I had no inclination to read.

On day 2 at home I did manage an eight-hour gap between doses of Codeine. I started taking Laxoll to help with the constipation but noticed no helpful effect. After a restless night with four (hopeful only) trips to the loo, I took a nap on my bed mid-afternoon.

Day 3 was lovely weather (late autumn in New Zealand) and I took my first walk outside to see my horse. I used the door that allowed me to take two smaller steps to exit the house, bracing my butt against the door frame and stepping down sideways, as illustrated earlier.

The back of my right foot still had the sore spot developed in the hospital. I experimented with ways to keep the back of the foot elevated, so it would not be touching the couch or bed when I was lying down. It was a small but nagging discomfort. Eventually, I used a bit of ribbon to tie a doubled-over thick woolly sock around my ankle to take the pressure off the sore spot.

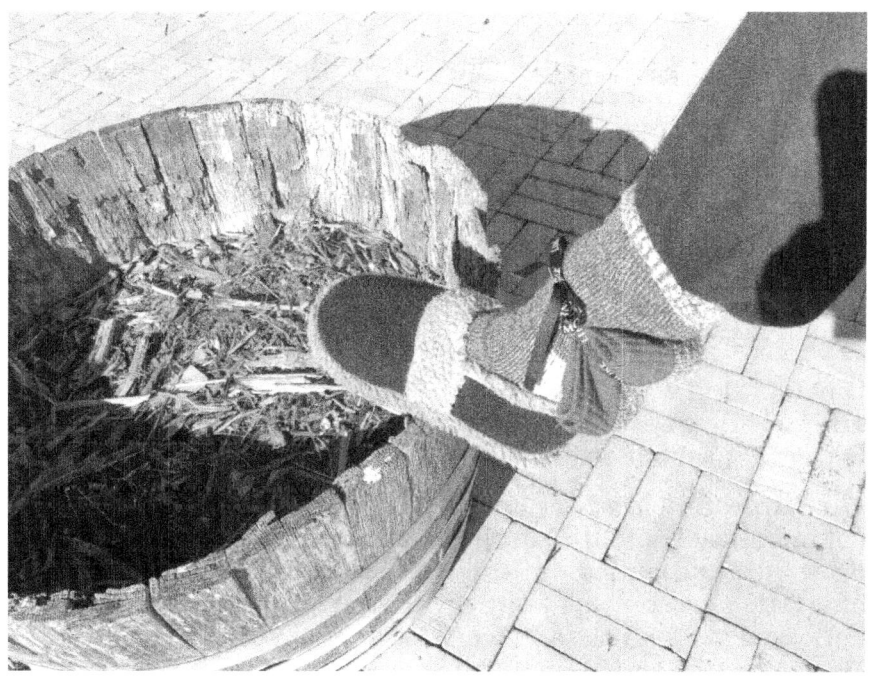

The back of my right heel developed a chronic sore spot. I tied a little pad of thick sock material around my ankle to help keep my heel raised off the surface my foot is resting on. I had one for day wear and one for sleeping. It was especially helpful for the first few weeks when I had to sleep on my back.

I managed to put in laundry and began to help organize the pantry of our new kitchen. I could walk around the house using just one crutch.

I was still getting up four times a night for an attempt at the loo and taking Laxoll in the hope of a bowel movement. Bowel relief was very slow in coming, and causing much discomfort, so it was a gold star moment when something finally happened.

By day 5 this week I could dress myself, other than putting on socks, which gave a nice feeling of achievement. I was also making more of my breakfast. Bryan still helped with moving hot things from A to B. I had my first shower at home, which went well. For the last few days I had used Baby Wipes to help keep clean.

I felt up to organising our plates and other dishes into the new kitchen cupboards. I was achieving close to a 90-degree bend with my right knee and keeping up with stepping high and pointing toes and stretching and gliding the feet under a chair on a plastic bag – the plastic bag shuffle. Music helped.

I could sit for a while at the computer to do emails. With two knees in repair mode, before I sat I had to ensure that there was always something sturdy to my right and left to push myself upright safely, plus have my crutches in easy reach.

Day 6 of this week I squeezed myself into the car for the 30-minute ride to get my stitches removed. The car ride was extremely uncomfortable.

The surgeon held my attention with questions and commentary while the nurse seamlessly removed the dressings and pulled out the stitches without my being aware of it. The surgeon was happy with how things looked and endorsed my keenness to work on my own physical therapy. He warned me again about the constipation problems with taking Codeine.

Getting back into the car, we had a bit of a misadventure. Bryan put my crutches in the back seat, then closed the back door, not realizing that my hand was still around the back-door jamb as I struggled to leverage myself into the car. I managed to squeak, "Fingers, Fingers!" and he quickly opened the door again.

Fortunately, the rubber door seal had taken most of the impact and my nails did not turn black. Poor Bryan felt terrible. It made a good story to tell for several days.

In the afternoon, I walked to our hayshed and then as far as the mailbox about 25 meters away. We have a large sealed driveway, on which I can walk circuits if I don't want to venture too far from home.

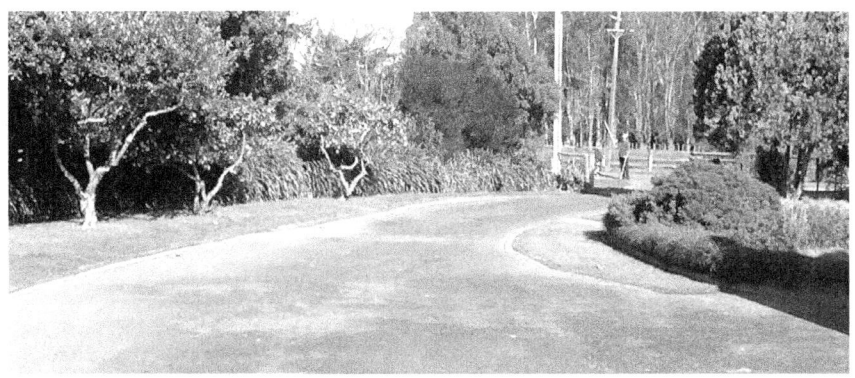

Raising my crutch in celebration the first time I made it to our mailbox.

Day 7, I walked morning and afternoon, going a bit further each time. My aim for next week is to cut the Codeine from every 8 hours to every 12 hours to help my digestive system return to some semblance of normality.

Summary of Achievements for Week 2

Day 8 since Operation

- Travel home by car was painful.

- Needed help with socks and shoes and getting up from couch.

- Surgeon recommended keeping legs up when not walking, to help counteract blood clots.

Day 9

Grateful for husband's help and company.

- Got onto and off couch independently as well as bed at night.
- Needed something to brace on to get up and my crutches had to be handy.
- Alternated reclining with legs up, sitting in a chair doing 'foot on plastic bag' exercise and walking around with my crutches.
- Had no desire to read. TV helped time pass. Mind was still fuzzy from the general anaesthetic, Codeine and Arcoxia.
- Bowels remained uncomfortable.
- Cut Codeine from 6-hourly to 8-hourly.

Day 10

- First walk outside gave me a mental boost.

Day 11

- Put on laundry, pottered briefly in the kitchen. Managed with one crutch at times.

Day 12

- Could finally put socks on by myself.
- Had first shower at home.
- Helped make my breakfast but not yet carrying hot items.
- Getting 90-degree bend in my right knee; left knee more reluctant.
- Could sit in a chair using the computer for a short time.

Day 13

- Had uncomfortable car trip (30 minutes) to have stiches removed.

- Walked 25 meters outside with crutches.

Day 14

- Took two outdoor walks with crutches. A bit further each time, maybe 50 meters.

NOTES:

NOTES:

Chapter 5: Week Three

This week I managed to dress myself fully including socks, made most of my own breakfast and did laundry.

We finally cleared the kitchen things out of much of the living room, which freed up a comfortable couch with a great view. I could put my legs up and contemplate the clouds.

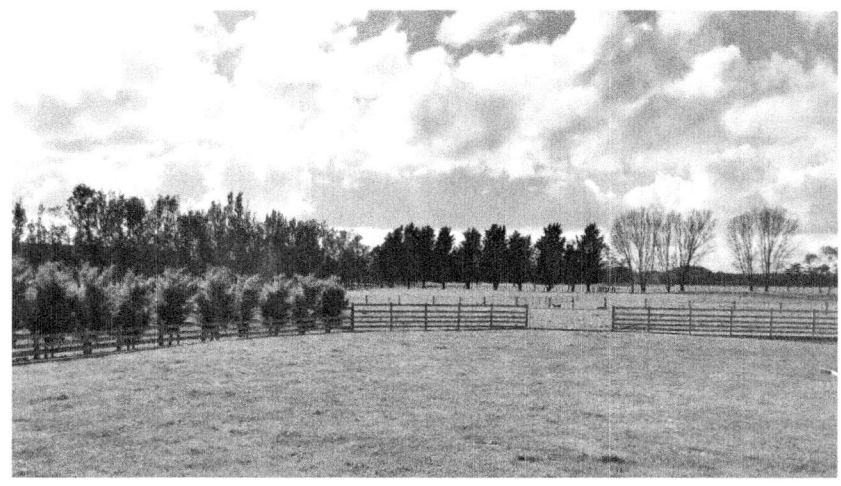

The view out the window from the living room couch.

My good friend, Bridget, came to visit on day 1 of this week. I made egg salad for our lunch. We visited my horse, Boots, so that Bridget could clean her feet. Bryan has taken over doing the horse chores, but his back is not up to cleaning horse feet. Bridget and I walked down the road for about 60 meters – my first walk away from home.

At the end of day 2, I decided to go cold turkey with the Codeine. It was playing havoc with my digestive system and the constipation was extreme.

It took the good part of a week for my system to return to a semblance of 'normal' as the gut microbes regained their mojo. The process included multiple pit stops over 24 hours and an overall lack of energy.

I ate kiwifruit and drank lots of liquids to help things along. I used adult incontinence undies for a day or two to catch any accidents, but there was only one accident. The special undies removed some of the strain of the situation because it took a while to get to the toilet. It was such an effort and took so long when I had to undress and dress again.

I did two short walks a day and occasionally snoozed in the afternoon or rested quietly. Taking a shower was exhausting. A 'plus' was that stopping the Codeine stopped the extreme dryness in my mouth.

On day 5 of this week I felt queasy, had little appetite and found it hard to keep warm. A walk in the afternoon left me sore. I presumed the last of the Codeine had worn off.

On a positive note, I felt inclined to do a bit of reading for the first time since the operation. Reading has always been one of my favorite activities. It was a worry to feel spaced out for so long.

Evidently a full anaesthetic can take a long time to clear from the system. I needed to remember that I had an epidural as well as a full anaesthetic. The brain can remain fuzzy for quite a while. Research reminded me that response to anaesthetics is also influenced by lifestyle elements like obesity, smoking, history of alcohol or drug use.

On the night leading to day 6, I got no sleep due to knee pain. In the morning I tried to manage the pain by walking a bit further than yesterday with the result that at least my head felt clearer.

On day 7, I managed to get one foot on a pedal of the Exercycle and rock it back and forth a little bit. The swelling in my legs was gradually subsiding. I massaged from ankle to thigh several times a day to help the fluid move along. When not walking or doing exercises, I kept my legs up to help decrease the swelling, as the surgeon had advised.

My appetite improved, and the bowels felt better. I interspersed 'legs up' with walking around the house and was enthused enough to make an apple crumble.

Summary of Achievements for Week Three

Day 15 Since Operation

- Made my own breakfast.
- Felt comfortable carrying hot things.
- Prepared lunch for a visiting friend.
- Walked with friend for 60 meters.

Day 16

Stopped Codeine cold-turkey due to severe constipation.

Day 17

- Dry mouth from Codeine was gone but I felt sore and below par generally as the last of the Codeine wore off.
- I finally felt like reading and less like a mental zombie.

Day 18

Two short walks each day.

Day 19

- Little appetite, felt queasy.
- Hard to keep warm.
- Very uncomfortable night due to knee pain.

Day 20

- Walked outside for fresh air to help clear my malaise.
- Twice daily, massaged from ankles upward to help reduce the swelling.

Day 21

- Right foot rocked exercycle pedal back and forth.
- Noticed obvious reduction of swelling.
- Appetite improved.
- Bowels felt better.
- Made an apple crumble, sitting to peel the apples.

NOTES:

Chapter 6: Weeks Four and Five

Reading became more enjoyable each day. I baked a batch of brownies, but it took me three separate sessions in the kitchen, putting up my legs between bouts of activity. At least I had a shiny new kitchen to do it in.

The new kitchen has lots of sliding drawers which replaced cupboards with doors and shelves. We were still experimenting with what fitted best in the new sliding drawers, which made finding a particular item rather engrossing.

This week I walked a little bit further each day and helped to prepare meals.

I've managed to turn myself in bed to lie on my left side for a short while. Each time I made the effort I could stay there a minute or so longer.

The top of my left thigh developed nerve pain. I regained my digestive health after stopping the Codeine, but at times the pain to pay for it was considerable. Level of comfort seemed to depend on how much I had expected of my knees.

It paid to remember that not only did the muscles surrounding my knees have to heal and adjust, but the rest of my body needed to re-organize itself to the new angles and the new way of moving. Every now and then my lower back and hips reminded me of this.

After two sleepless nights, I took a Paracetamol (Tylenol) to dull the knee pain so I could sleep a little bit. The plan was to take these only when I couldn't get to sleep any other way.

When I did a lot of walking around the house doing chores, it was a good idea to cut down on my outdoor walking. Most days, I added another twenty metres to my walks down the road. Sitting in a chair at the computer was still painful, but I tried to build several bursts of it into each day.

On day 6 of this week, I decided to use ice packs on my knees at bedtime, rather than begin to depend more on the Paracetamol. Icing is an interesting topic because the recuperating muscle cells need body temperature to keep blood flowing freely. Since the blood brings the oxygen necessary for repair, and removes the waste products of metabolism, applying ice slows down all these processes.

The ice did help dull the pain and allowed me to relax enough so that when I pulled the ice packs off after about twenty minutes, I could usually sleep for a few hours.

Week Four

This week I intensified my knee bending efforts. My horse's sand arena contains a set of rails lying on the ground. I devised an exercise where I placed one foot on a rail, paused, then stepped that foot over the rail. I used my crutches at first, then later my walking poles, for support.

Once the first foot was across the rail, I tried my best to lift the second foot straight up and onto the rail. At first this was devilishly hard, and I cheated by swinging the foot sideways to bring it up onto the rail.

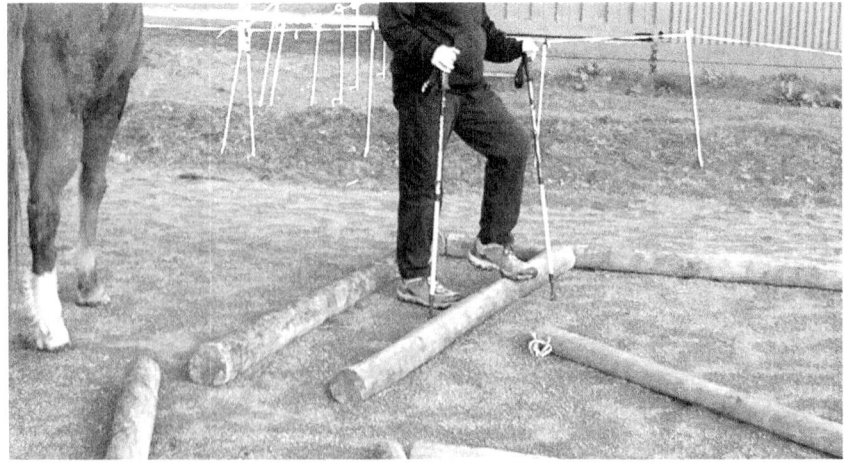

I've put one foot up on a rail and am playing with the bend in the knee.

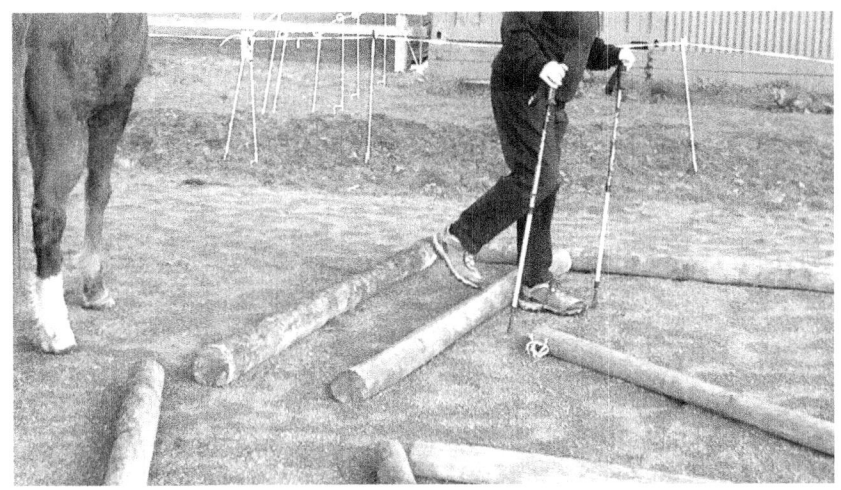

I'm lifting the second foot up and forward to sit on the rail. At first this was hard and painful, so I swung my foot sideways to set it onto the rail.

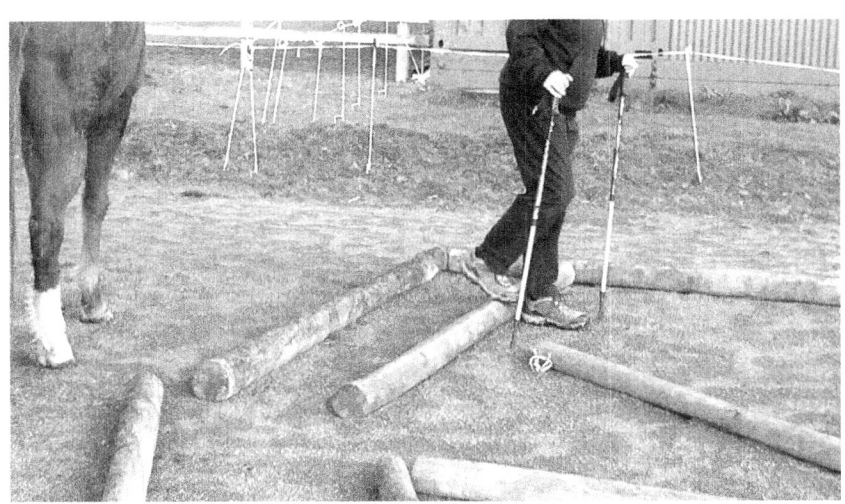

I'm resting the second foot up on the rail. By shifting my torso weight backward or forward, I could increase or decrease the pressure on the knee resting on the rail.

I had about twelve of these rails to navigate and began to faithfully do them at least once each day. It was much more fun having a series of obstacles to negotiate than to do endless repeats with one piece of gear.

Almost imperceptibly, over the next five weeks, it became easier and easier. By Week 9, I no longer had to swing my second foot sideways. The flexibility of the left knee consistently lagged behind that of the right knee. I also set up two higher rails to keep working on lifting the second foot up higher, but it took a while to manage it without swinging the second foot sideways.

My tax-return deadline loomed, so it was time to get my brain into gear. My mind still felt as if it was not yet running at full throttle. At one point I had to use simple algebra to work out one of the numbers needed on my tax return. I knew that I knew how to do it. I even remembered the teacher who taught us basic algebra. I stared at the task and tried various options for half an hour. Finally, I cracked it, just before giving up and calling my daughter-in-law for help.

Years ago, I took on trimming Boots' feet, doing a little bit often so it never got to be a big chore. I trimmed right before the operation, but after five weeks I found a person to do it for me. Unfortunately, she trimmed out the heels, which left a bad feeling. I had printed out pictures and explained how I wanted it done, but I obviously wasn't clear enough.

Being winter, Boots got hay every day at noon, which gave me a reason to go out and walk. We usually spent time doing activities that didn't need me to walk around much. She was very conscious that I was compromised in my movement.

A couple of times this week, I worked Boots around me on a long rope. I walked a small inner circle while she walked and trotted a large circle around me.

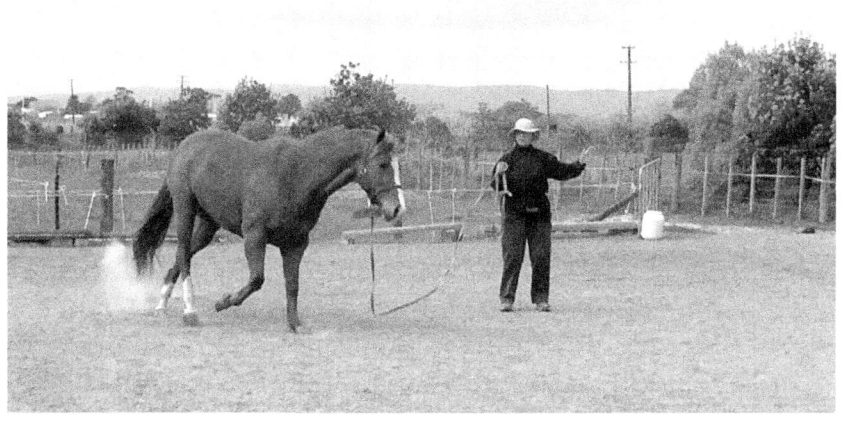

During week five I was able to ask Boots to do more active exercise on a long rein. I can remain quiet in the center while she works around me.

Week Five

During week five I went online and purchased a few Kindle books about recovering from knee replacement. Perhaps I should have done this sooner, ideally before the operation. The books set out a nice variety of exercises, some of which I added to my repertoire.

YouTube also had a few helpful videos. Due to the agony of driving into town, I opted to do my own physio rather than have 'appointments' for which one is warned to take pain medication to 'get the most out of them'.

My therapy approach was little and often, listening to what my body told me. Little and often is the way I work to develop new skills and maintain flexion in my horse. Reading the knee replacement books encouraged me to become more robust with my physical therapy.

If you have the time and inclination, it is probably a good idea to read some of these books and watch relevant videos before the operation and learn to do the exercises as much as wonky knees allow. Had I not been immersed in our kitchen renovation, I would probably have done that.

Most of the books are written by physical therapists who have not had knee replacements. What also made me uneasy about physical therapists is that they work via 'appointments'. They see each client for a short while and no doubt feel they must earn their money by 'getting a lot done' during each session. Hence the warnings to be sure to take your pain medication an hour before each physical therapy session.

It may also be easy to believe that physical therapy appointments are 'enough' and not carry on with lots of short repeats throughout the day, even though this is highly recommended. Another danger is that a 'session' with the therapist might create so much pain that one is averse to doing more for quite a while.

The exercises themselves are not rocket science. The keys are:

- working to increase the bend.
- straighten the leg if it is not straight.
- gradually increase walking distance.
- improve balance.

The more creative ways I could find to do these things frequently during the day, the less onerous the whole process. At the back of the book is a list of the exercises I found helpful.

Once I got going, I didn't find walking super painful. However, encouraging a greater angle of bend varied from painful to excruciating. I tried to learn to smile through the pain rather than grimace. Much easier to talk about than to do. Smiling and breathing with the pain helps the muscles relax into the new shape.

In her book, *Fast Track Your Recovery from a Total Knee Replacement,* Michelle Stiles, a physiotherapist, suggested working mainly on getting the bend during the first three weeks while still on pain medication, then later focussing on walking distance and other weight-bearing exercises. I can't quite imagine how I would have been able to do that. Maybe it makes more sense with a single knee replacement.

As the swelling reduced, I increased the massage pressure around the knee. I massaged with my hands and also used a wee three-pronged vibrating gadget.

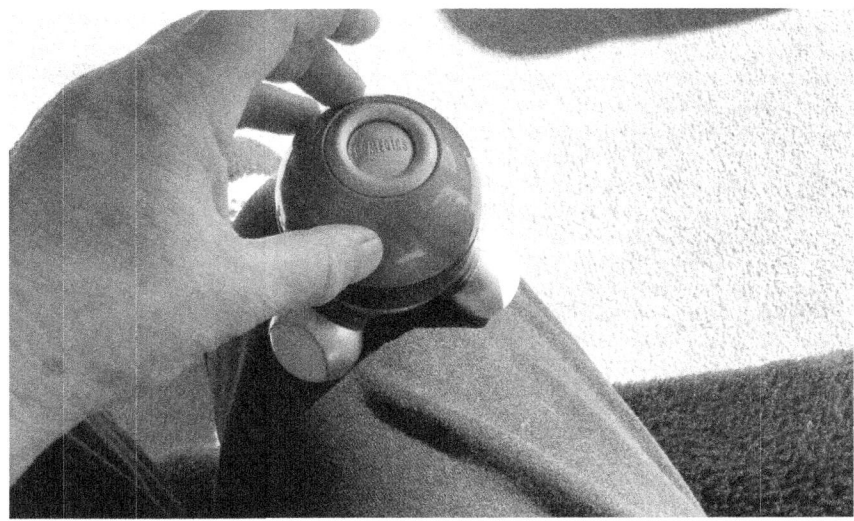

This gadget sends out a strong vibration that stimulates the muscle tissue, creating a tingling feeling. As healing progressed, I used it closer to the knee.

Summary for Weeks Four and Five

- Carried on with morning walks, adding distance most days.

- Read several books & watched video clips, authored by physiotherapists, about recovery from total knee replacement.

- Engaged more with mental activities such as playing Scrabble against the computer.

- Intensified my knee-bending exercises to three or more sessions per day.

- Sought out new places to do creative knee-bending exercises.

- Added horse activities at mid-day.

- Used vibrating gadget to stimulate the muscles around the knees.

- Did more meal preparation.

NOTES:

Chapter 7: Weeks Six and Seven

Week Six

It soon became apparent that recovery was not a strictly linear process. There were good days and not-so-good days. During this week I enjoyed a walk first thing in the morning after getting up. The aim continued to be to go a bit further each day, but I didn't castigate myself if the legs suggested that a shorter walk was in order.

While walking I carried light-weight walking poles held horizontally so I could swing my arms naturally. Walking was still slow. I raised my knees as much as I could. I used my poles when traffic made me move to the slanting side of road. The last thing I wanted was to twist a knee or have a fall. The poles were also handy when the new puppy down the road ran out to jump up and say hello. If the legs got tired, I used the poles putting as little pressure on them as possible.

Moving from my couch to sitting in a recliner chair was an interesting process. There is an air gap between my recliner foot rest when it is up, and the seat. My knees lie across this gap. Being used to the support of the couch, the knees quickly began to complain, and I had to return to the couch after about ten minutes. I think this is a good exercise to stretch and strengthen muscles behind the knees.

Some physiotherapists suggest a similar exercise sitting in one chair and putting the feet up on another chair.

Each evening, I sat in the recliner until it became too uncomfortable. It was a couple of weeks before I could give up the couch altogether.

Week Seven

I started to put considerably more effort into regular short 'knee bend' workouts. Outside I found all the things in my horse arena, and around the yard, onto which I could lift a foot and practice bending just a tiny bit more than last time.

I did a few bends at one obstacle, then walked to the next one. This spread the bending load. I found this method so much easier than continuous repeats in one place to the point of extreme discomfort. The walking in between the bending repeats gave the muscles time to have a think and regroup.

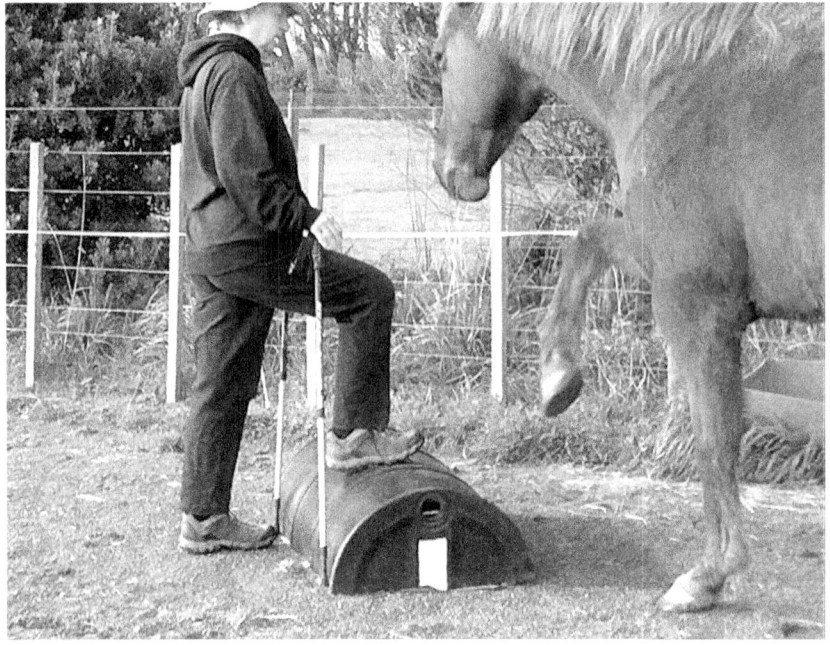

Boots is helping me with my knee-bending exercises.

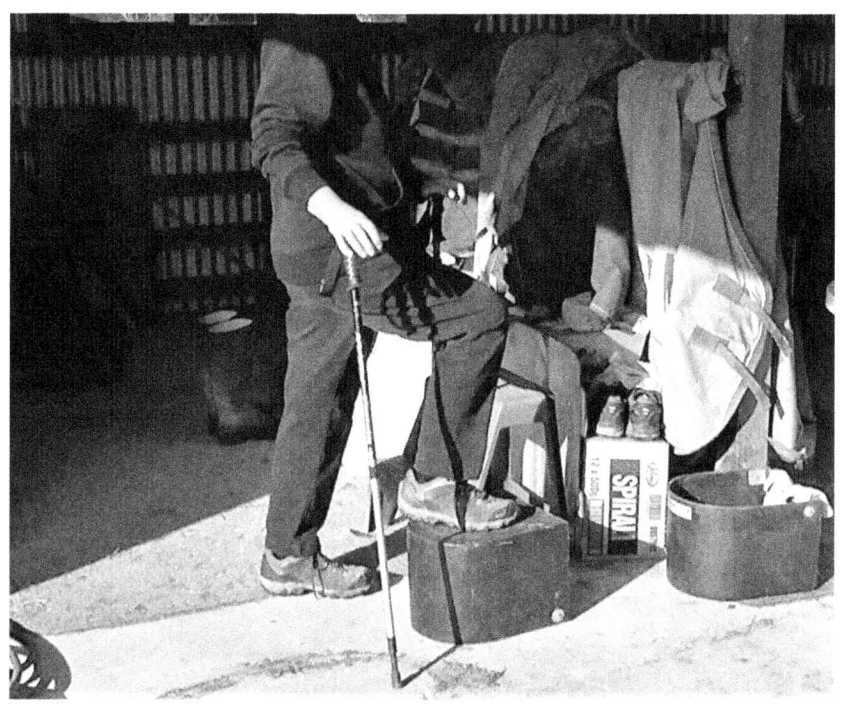

By tilting my weight forward over my knee, I could gradually induce more of a bend. Using the poles assured my balance.

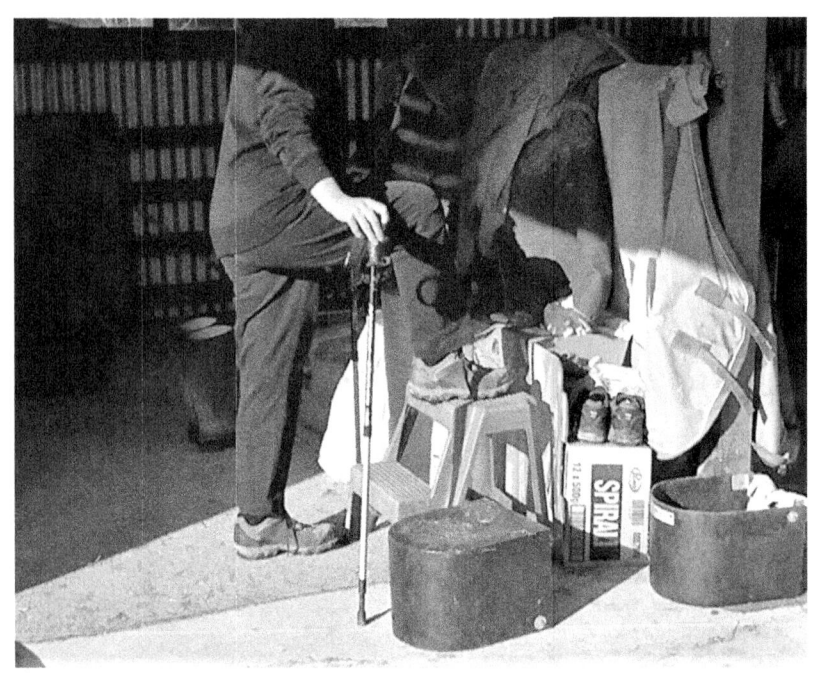

Each object I used gave me a different challenge.

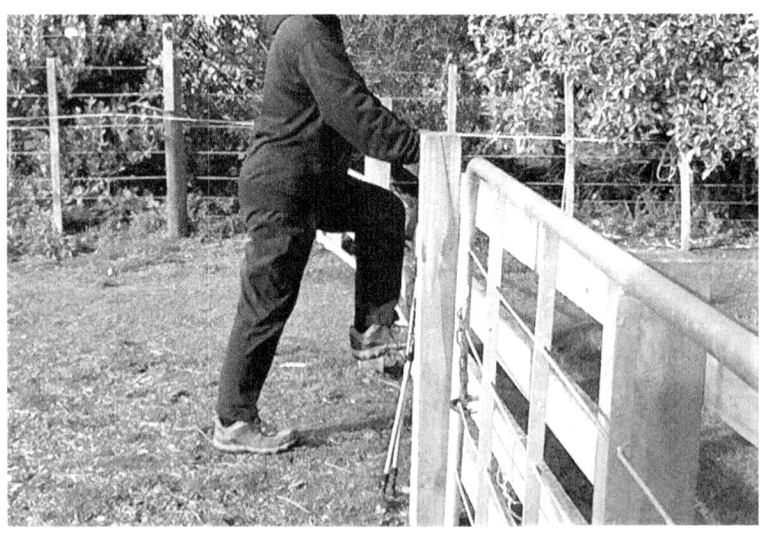

Fences turned out to be useful. Here I can do a knee bend and a calf-stretch. Eventually I was able to put my foot on the next board up.

In the house, I set up another circuit of 'stations'. I expanded my exercise repertoire to take in the hall where I could do marching, walking sideways, walking backwards and 'lunging' type steps.

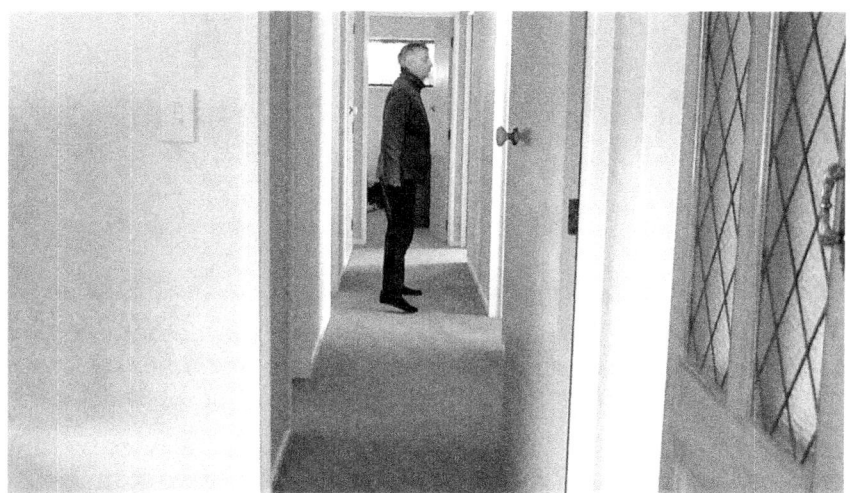

Using the hallway to walk sideways and backwards, do marching and lunging steps. This was especially helpful during wet weather.

The kitchen benchtop was handy for doing calf stretches, marching on the spot, the 'kick the butt' exercise, swinging a leg to the side, shallow squats and heel-to-toe exercises.

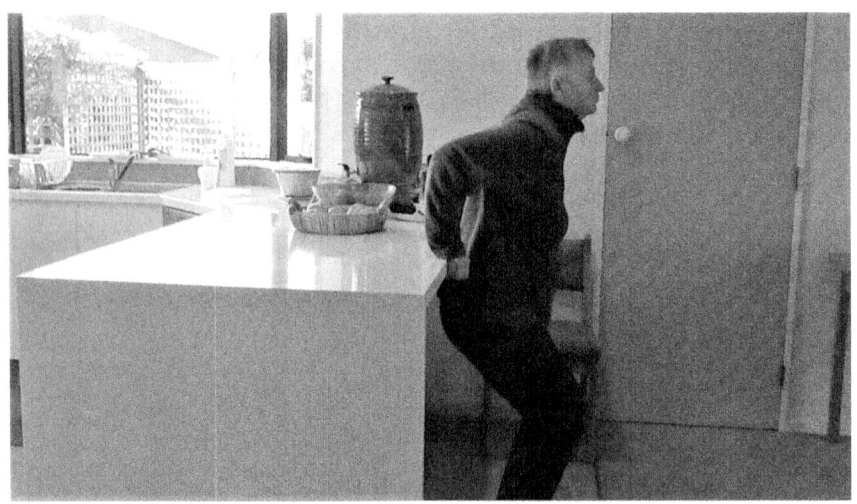

I used the kitchen bench for a variety of knee-bending exercises. Here I dropped my weight down to cause the knees to bend. I also did this standing against a wall.

On day 1 of this week, I woke up from a sound sleep and the weather was glorious, so I went for a half-hour walk both morning and late afternoon, with a shorter outing at noon when I fed my horse. Expecting to sleep well after so much activity, it was disappointing when sleep eluded me.

It seemed that when I got a good night's sleep, I tended to overdo exercise the following day, especially when it was bright and sunny.

Day 2 included a lot of knee bending exercises and two shorter walks. I also managed to clean all four of my horse's feet, which I do as often as I can because the wet winter paddocks often cause a fungal infection in horses' feet. Day 2 ended with a second night of very little sleep.

Day 3, I walked and worked on knee-bending. For the first time ever, I developed a throbbing pain in my right (better) knee that did not calm down when I put my legs up. Ice helped dull the pain, so I iced when I went to bed and took Paracetamol for the fifth time since coming home from the hospital. Slept a bit, woke up to the pain still there, so iced some more and managed to sleep again.

By morning the pain had eased but both scars felt extra stiff and tight. I spent time in the horse arena walking over rails and later helped my daughter-in-law clean Boots' feet and I managed a bit of maintenance on one of her feet. I hoped I can soon do a little bit often. A visit from the family brightened up our Sunday morning.

It was a new milestone when I got both feet on the pedals of the exercycle and initiated a bit of back-and-forth movement. Books I've read cautioned against too much too early with an exercycle. It is all a balance between doing enough to keep the scar tissue at bay without setting up extra inflammation by doing too much.

Day 4 followed a night with some sleep, but legs felt sore and restless. Lying on my left side was not comfortable. I gave the muscles an especially good massage while getting dressed.

I tended Boots' front feet after playing a few games with her. When I put my legs up for a rest after being outdoors, it became easier to rest for longer in the recliner chair. I could sit with my knees bent, as in the photo, for up to 80 seconds.

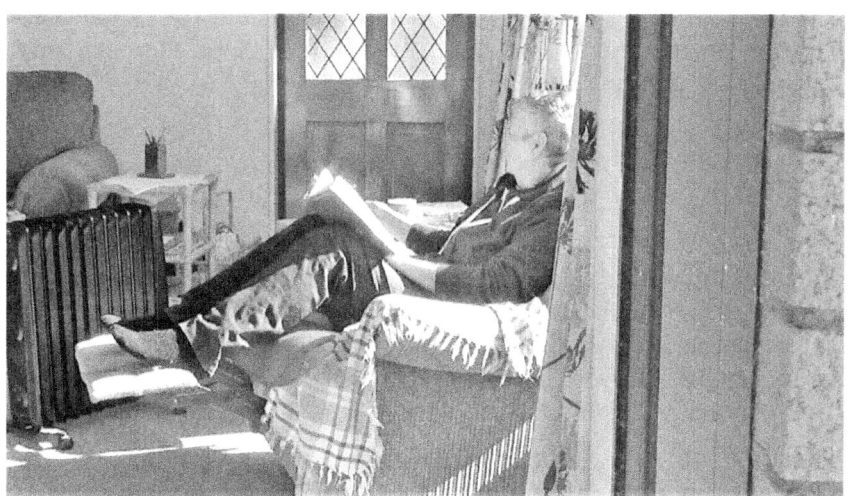

By setting my heels against the footrest, I maintained close to a 90-degree bend in my knees. Over the weeks, this gradually became easier and maintained longer.

Comfort while sitting in a chair at the computer was improving, but it was important to get up frequently to walk the stiffness out of the knees, so they wouldn't seize up.

I accompanied Bryan for grocery shopping for the first time since the operation. It was the first car outing since my post-op check-up back in week two. I felt more comfortable in the car but wouldn't like to go much further than the 20-minute trip into town. I managed the supermarket but was relieved to sit down after walking the aisles.

I was in the process of learning how to use my walking poles in the proper Nordic style. I found that my knees felt relatively comfortable striding out and forward, helped by the swinging motion of the shoulders and supported by the poles.

To find out more about Urban or Nordic Poling. The web address is www.urbanpoling.com. The health benefits from this type of exercise are considerable. More knee surgeons are becoming aware of how helpful it can be for their patients.

Day 5: I had a reasonable sleep last night. We took a trip into town that included three stops plus crossing streets heavy with traffic. Using my walking poles gave me a bit of security because it showed people that I was going to be slower than the average pedestrian.

It was also a good lesson in just how unfriendly city sidewalks can be for anyone with a movement handicap. There were funny steps and ledges and uneven pavements everywhere.

Even my small local library has an undulating floor which surprised me. Before my operation I had never noticed the unevenness. I think the community is so relieved that the library is still allowed to exist, that they are not going to worry about an uneven floor.

It's nice to have regained the confidence to go out and about, although I'm a country girl and usually prefer staying at home.

Day 6: Sleep last night was reasonable again. Several times I managed to lie on my left side slightly longer than before. In an early morning frost, I took my longest walk yet, using my poles in the Nordic Walking style most of the way. Today we took two trips into town, one for my second check-up with the surgeon.

The surgeon was happy. As soon as he saw me walking to his office, he said my knee function was looking excellent for a double knee replacement. He checked the degree of bend in a cursory manor by seeing how I sat in a chair. He liked the idea of Nordic walking. Unless a problem arose, the surgeon would see me again in a year's time. At that point he would organize x-rays to give us a baseline to compare with any changes in the future.

My right knee had always been better, and I was getting over 90 degrees with it. The left knee was a bit more recalcitrant. The surgeon said they look for 90 degrees at 7-8 weeks for a double replacement. I knew it was in my court to keep up the exercises to maintain steady progress.

I asked the surgeon about how the memory of my previous walking alignment, held by my old shoes, might affect the balance of my new knees. He agreed that changing the insoles or investing in new shoes was a good idea. I organized to buy a new pair of walking shoes.

The other trip to town was to get my new iPad set up by the store's technical person. After an hour of standing and concentrating I felt faint in the heat of the store. I stripped off extra clothes and put my head between my knees for a few minutes and was soon feeling better. I should have asked to switch to their lower desk where we could have sat down. The faintness came over suddenly and surprised me as I don't have a history of fainting.

Later in the day I felt the results of the morning's exertion in the rest of my body. It's a continuing challenge to do as many stretch exercises as possible without setting up more inflammation. Sometimes it feels necessary to ease up and give other parts of the body time to catch up with the new alignment.

Summary for Weeks Six and Seven

- Walked more.
- Was diligent with knee-bending exercises at least twice daily with odd ones thrown in throughout the day.
- Cleaned horse's feet for the first time.
- Managed to get both feet onto the exercycle pedals and rock them back and forth (not yet a full turn).
- Regularly sat in recliner chair with legs bent for up to 80 seconds.
- Worked at computer in 20-minute segments.
- Learned how to do proper Nordic Walking with my poles.
- First outing to supermarket with Bryan.
- First outing (with Bryan) into town with multiple stops.
- Second check-up with surgeon.

NOTES:

Chapter 8: Weeks Eight and Nine

Week Eight

Overall, sleeping was getting easier. I even had occasional dreams. Sometimes I was able to doze off for a while lying on my left side, which has long been my favorite sleeping side. Each night lying on my side remained comfortable for slightly longer.

I stopped using ice at bedtime because icing slows down blood flow and all the things cells need to do to repair. I guess the idea is to slow down formation of scar tissue but speed up the process of the stretchy muscles repairing themselves.

Sleep was still interrupted with going to the toilet two or three times a night as well as having to wake up each time I wanted to shift position.

I walked every day it wasn't raining. I usually walked first thing after getting up, again at noon, doing my outdoor knee bend course, plus a shorter walk in the late afternoon. I tried to clean out at least two of Boots' feet most days and do a bit of rasping on the underside. It felt like I would soon be able to put at least her front feet on the hoof stand so I could rasp the toes.

This week I continued to alternate sitting at my computer with walking to stretch the knees. Every now and then I reclined on the couch to read or reflect.

Half way through the week, I was able to put Boots' front feet on the hoof stand and do some trimming. I'm sticking with one foot per day. I also made a short horse-training video to demonstrate a haltering method, in answer to someone's on-line question.

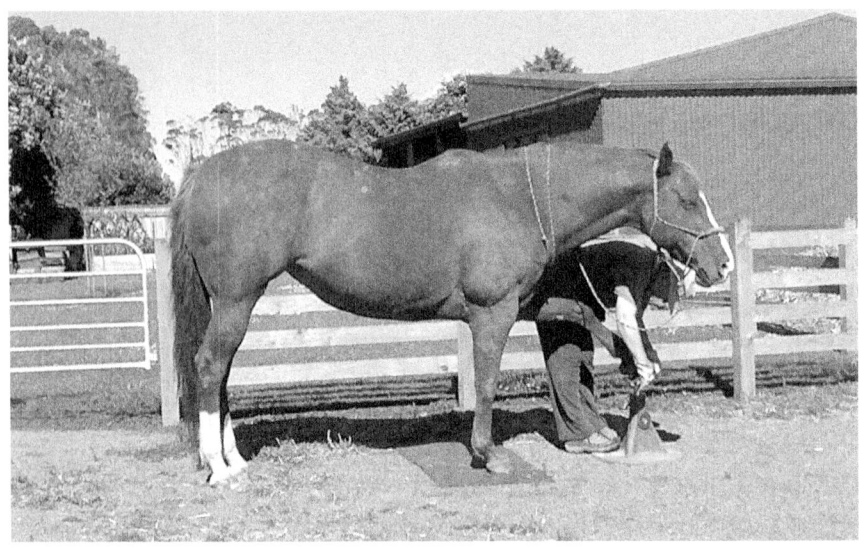

Boots co-operates nicely to have her foot on the hoof stand.

I now regularly got both feet on the pedals of the exercycle and could rotate them back and forth for a few minutes. The right knee was almost ready to do a full revolution but would have to wait for the left knee to catch up. I used the exercycle after I'd been walking so the knees were already warmed up.

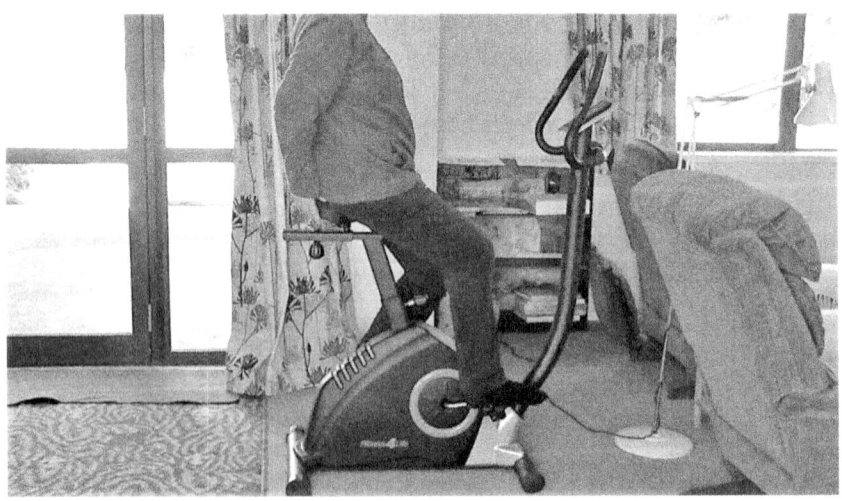

It took a while to get both feet on the exercycle pedals. Getting on and off was tricky because I didn't want to twist anything.

Bryan and I both had nasty head colds this week, but I tried hard to keep up the flexion exercises. The real test was the floor-polishing task, where I flexed my knee as far as possible under a chair sitting on a smooth floor. I wore woolly socks to reduce the friction as much as possible. It helped to mark, on a strip of masking tape, how much further back I could pull my toes each day. There is nothing like good bio-feedback to keep up motivation.

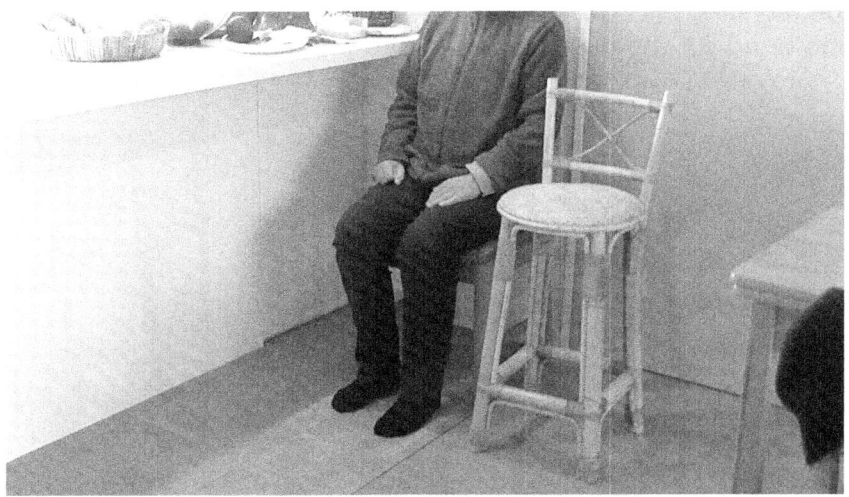

This is a slightly more sophisticated version of sliding the foot back and forth on a plastic bag. Woolly socks slipped easily on the vinyl floor. The masking tape alongside my feet allowed me to mark how far back under the chair I could slide each foot. This method meant I could actually measure each knee's increased bending ability. Having the marks on the tape was strong motivation to push through the resistance and do a bit more than last time. I used the stool and the counter-top to pull myself up from the chair.

I was now able to sit for longer in a recliner chair. How easy or hard it was to keep my knees bent tucked against the footrest gave me a good indication of how supple (or not) things were at that point in time.

The car trip into town for groceries felt a little more comfortable. It was still uncomfortable cruising the supermarket aisles. I think if I had to drive, I could.

During days 6 and 7 of this week the knees were quite stiff. Maybe being run-down with a cold was part of the reason. I kept up my basic exercise routines. Maybe the soreness was related to holding the knees bent for longer while sitting in my recliner. I had added this to my other regular bending exercises. My new accomplishment this week was navigating the big step into the house without a crutch. I only needed one hand on the door frame as I stepped up.

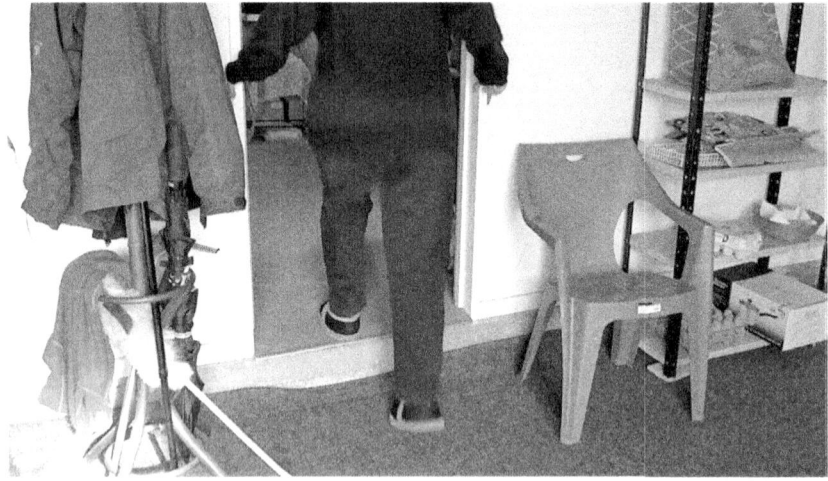

Stepping straight up the 20-centimetre high (7.8 inches) step that leads into the main parts of our house. I used hands on the door frame to give me more confidence. Previously I stepped up and down sideways using my crutches and later one of my poles. The maximum height for steps generally is 7 inches, so this step is extra-high.

Week Nine

I started week nine with a nice long walk with my Nordic poles, as it was a beautiful day. I was getting better at alternating active movement with 'legs up' for reading, perusing my iPad or playing Scrabble against the computer.

Between rests, I fitted in bursts of housework like vacuuming and baking and horse work outside. Whenever I was outside, I used my outdoor exercise gadgets. At least once a day I noted my progress on the exercycle. I couldn't yet do a full revolution, but the possibility was edging closer. All these activities were interspersed with working at my computer sitting in a chair.

Occasionally I walked a little bit on the moist and uneven lawn. Lawn-walking was much more challenging than walking on flat pavement. It brought home to me how much my original knees gave me 'independent suspension' to move on uneven ground. While I helped with horse chores each afternoon I had to walk on sticky, pugged-up paddock surfaces. I went slowly, with my poles for support, and took care to not twist anything.

The knees still felt very tight whenever I changed from sitting at my computer to standing and walking.

This week I managed to bake a batch of cookies without having to do it in stages with resting my knees in-between. I think it is important to notice all these small changes. All the small changes together added up to much more freedom of movement and comfort.

During this week I continued to navigate the big step into the house squarely by lightly holding one side of the doorframe to give me assurance. After a few days doing this, I could walk up the step without holding on to anything. But I was careful to err on the side of caution. Getting too cocky could result in a twist or stumble.

The night of Day 4 was rough because a strong pain developed in the top of my right thigh. It was intrusive enough to stop me sleeping, so I took Paracetamol, which allowed me a few hours' rest. It felt like a pulled muscle. Maybe it was brought on by the stretching during Nordic walking.

Perhaps, when I manoeuvred to lie on my left side, I pulled the right knee up and strained it that way. It felt better in the morning and the pain only resurfaced vaguely during my morning walk. I managed to walk a little bit further than yesterday, which always gave a mental boost.

This week I realized that I could put on my undies standing up, as long as I balanced on the edge of my bed with the other hand. Another Week Nine milestone was stepping straight down a step leading into the house. Previously I had navigated the step-down sideways.

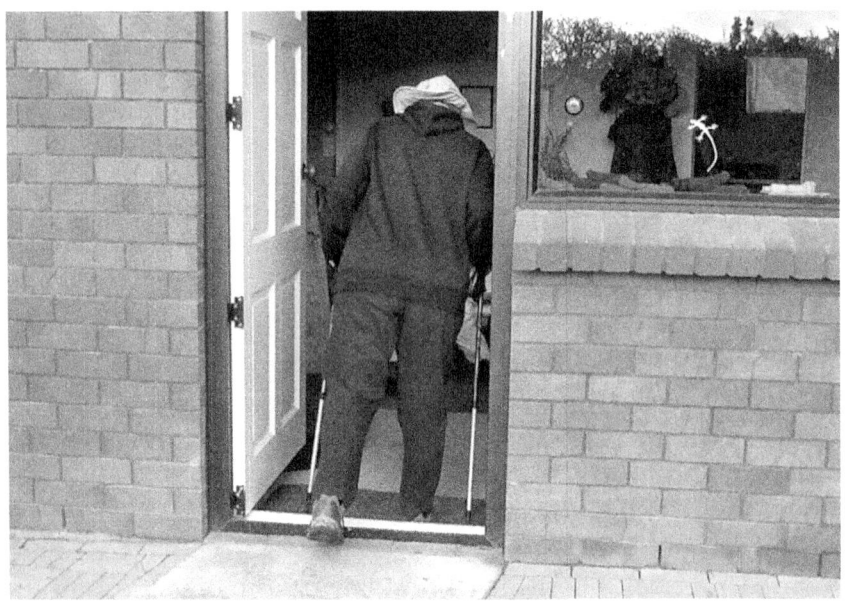

It was a milestone to be able to step straight down this step. There is an aluminium lip in front of my left foot, which made the whole thing a bit tricky. Until now I had navigated this step sideways, as shown in the next picture.

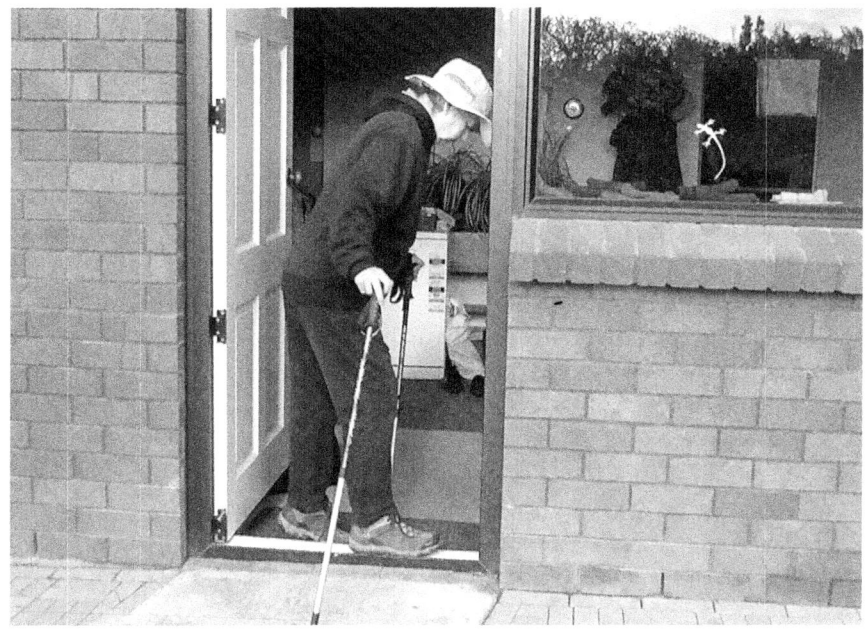

Sideways navigation of the step-down into the house.

By the end of this week, I could sleep soundly lying on my left side and just started to snooze briefly lying on my right side. The morning walk has become about one kilometre long. I stuck with that distance for a while until the knees arrived home a little less exhausted.

Summary for Weeks Eight and Nine

- Sleeping was easier, and I could lie on my left side by the end of week 9.
- Was able to do a bit more housework like vacuuming.
- Experimented daily with two feet on the exercycle pedals: full revolutions not yet possible.
- Managed a few more activities with the horse.
- Set up a chair with tape on the vinyl to measure and mark each day's bending capability for each knee.
- Experienced considerable stiffness after demanding more from knees.

- Stepped up the major step into house without a crutch for support.
- Stepped straight down a step into the house, rather than having to go down sideways (still with crutch or stick support).
- Began walking on uneven, soft lawn with stick support.
- Baked biscuits (cookies) without needing to pause for rests.
- Could put on undies standing up.
- Main morning walk distance increased to one kilometre.

NOTES:

Chapter Nine: Weeks Ten to Twelve

Week Ten

On Day 1 of this week, I found it a bit much to do a long early morning walk as well as walk a fair distance in the city. Day 2, I overdid my bending exercises, so by day three things were sore. Obviously, I'm still struggling to get the DOING-RESTING balance right.

The highlight of day 2 was a full backward rotation on the exercycle with my right knee. It came as a surprise as I was playing with the pedals. I generally tested my exercycle ability after our evening outdoor chores when the body and knees were already warmed up.

Day 3, I managed to work out what I had actually done on the exercycle to achieve the full rotation and repeated it twice. I didn't want to push my luck. I tried to work out how much the left knee still had to improve until it could also do a full rotation. Had to take Paracetamol (Tylenol) in the middle of the night to get back to sleep.

Stiff and sore on Day 4. Walked my maximum distance in the morning but took it easy in the afternoon.

A highlight of Week Ten, which only someone who has had two new knees will truly appreciate, was getting up from the toilet (and firm chairs) without bracing on anything. Sitting down was a bit harder, but possible with a support on one side.

Week Eleven

This week began with a walk that took me five rural fence posts further than yesterday's walk.

I was sitting relatively comfortably at my computer for longer. I put my timer across the room, so I had to get up to turn it off, making me walk every 20 minutes.

At this point I was wondering how long it would take before the knees stopped feeling like foreign objects. I thought it was a good question for the Facebook knee replacement group, but I didn't receive more than a couple of comments. Such groups are interesting but can be both a comfort and a worry.

On day 1 of this week, I managed a full revolution pedalling backwards with both knees. It felt like a major breakthrough. However, things were painful the next day, so I did less for a couple of days.

On Day 4, I took pain relief before my bout of exercises and managed four good backward rotations with just the right knee. But I didn't like the idea of medicating to push through the exercises.

My new Urban Poling poles arrived from Canada. They are nicer than the ones I can get in New Zealand. They have little angled rubber feet that are silent on the pavement. My other poles are ideal for off-road. I carried on with periods of walking on grass this week. It felt different and required continuous minor adjustment through the knees because the ground was not flat.

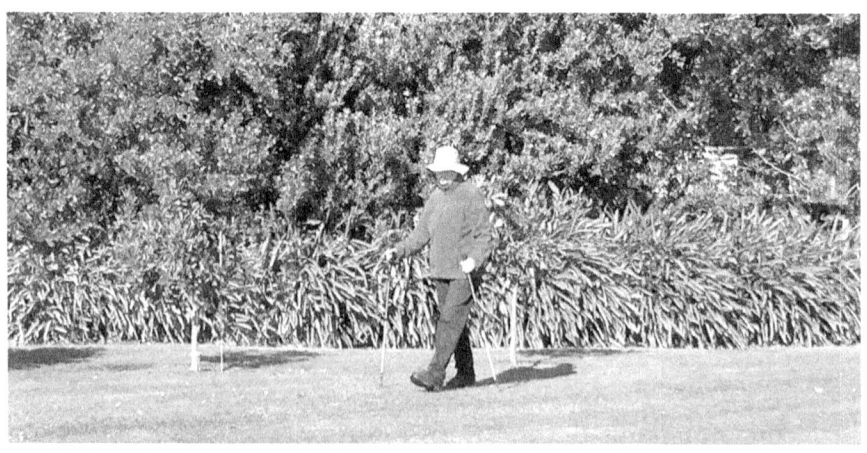

Walking on grass showed me just how much adjustment the knee and surrounding muscles make to cope with an uneven and less firm surface. It felt very different to walking on pavement.

Day 5 showed me that forcing the issue with the exercycle caused tightening muscles and more discomfort. I needed to keep listening to what the knees were saying and not get too keen to achieve a target for the sake of achieving it. Patience continued to be a virtue.

Day 7 and I did not heed my own advice. I must have pushed the walking, bending and exercycle a bit far yesterday. I forced my left knee to do two full backward rotations on the exercycle, to accompany my right knee. Both knees were seized up the next day. I probably needed to cut back to one daily exercycle session again.

During this week I became confident enough to light the fire by myself. It was mid-winter and on the occasional wet, windy drab day a cosy fire is a great comfort.

Week Twelve

This week continued my ongoing struggle with doing too much, ending up unusually sore and causing a day of doing less. I experimented with knee-bending exercises followed by exercycle twice a day. Some sessions on the exercycle allowed a complete backward rotation of either the right or left knee, but I'm not forcing it. I want to stay under the threshold of 'break out' pain.

I enjoyed using the new Urban Poling poles and extending my walking distance. Handling the poles as intended involved use of all the upper body muscles. What probably happened was that my enthusiastic use of the poles had exercised my upper body muscles to an unaccustomed level, so I had lactic acid stiffness all over, with the ensuing apathy toward more exercise.

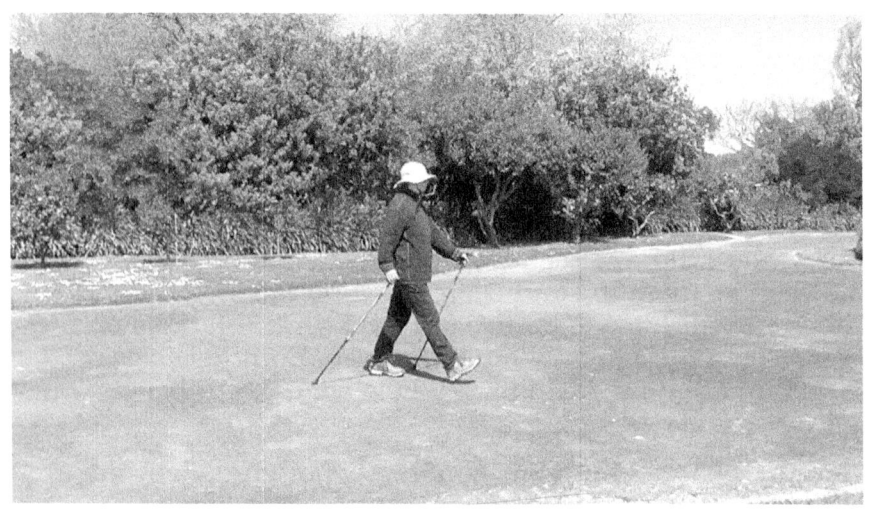

*Using my new Urban Poling poles. The support of the poles
makes it much easier to stride out and build a good rhythm.*

Sleep was generally much improved, despite waking twice
most nights to seek the toilet, plus the occasional part-
waking to change position. I could now manage two steps
into the house carrying firewood, without having to hold on
to the door frame. Stepping up was good, stepping down in a
'normal' manner will take longer to accomplish.

On day 5 of this week I woke up with a pulled muscle along
the outer edge of my left hand. I may have wrenched it while
bracing on it to change position in bed. I carried one pole in
my good hand during my morning walk, which encouraged
me to walk 'normally' rather than using two poles. It was
slower, but I was happy with the distance and how it all felt.

It also felt okay to do my knee-bending exercises outside with
just one pole to help maintain my balance.

On day 7 my hand felt better but I decided to do my morning
walk without the Urban Poles for a while to encourage a
'normal' walking gait. My walking still looked and felt zombie-
like. I was pleased with my distance which was almost as far
as I had gone with the poles.

After bending exercises, the right knee managed five backward half-rotations on the exercycle, each paired with a forward half-rotation because the left knee was still reluctant to take part in full revolutions.

With the right knee improved, getting the left knee to play along gave me a clear goal to strive for. The right knee was able to repeat the exercise after my late afternoon walking and bending exercises.

Summary for Weeks Ten to Twelve

- Right knee managed its first full backward rotation on the exercycle.
- Able to get up from firm chairs and toilet without bracing on something.
- Managed full backward rotations on the exercycle with both knees, although the left knee is still marginal.
- Organized firewood and fire without help.
- Slept better.
- Extended walking distance.
- Began walking further on the road without using poles.
- Right knee accomplished five forward and five backward rotations on the exercycle.

NOTES:

Chapter 10: Weeks Thirteen to Twenty

Week Thirteen

Walking without poles went well, but I still wanted the benefit of an upper body workout using the Nordic Walking poles. I decided to hold my poles horizontally on the outward journey to develop my 'normal' walking gait. On the return journey, I used my poles. The upper body engagement was strongly apparent when I used the poles correctly in the Nordic style.

I managed a second day of right knee full backward rotations on the exercycle. I worked hard to avoid a relapse into breakout pain for this task.

On day 3, I reached a major milestone. I walked all the way to the stopbank (levee) at the nearby river, including the climb up to the top of the levee, a roundtrip distance of about 2 km.

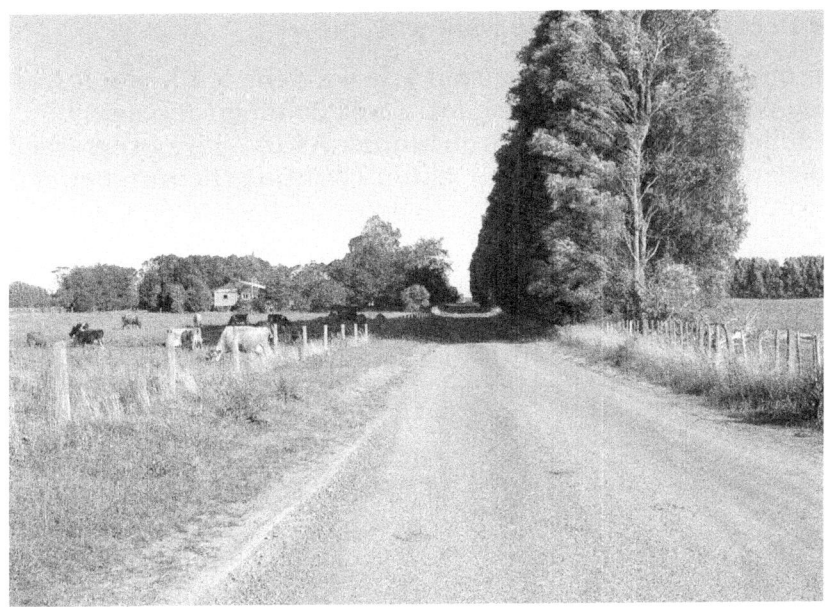

The road between our house and the river -a favorite walk.

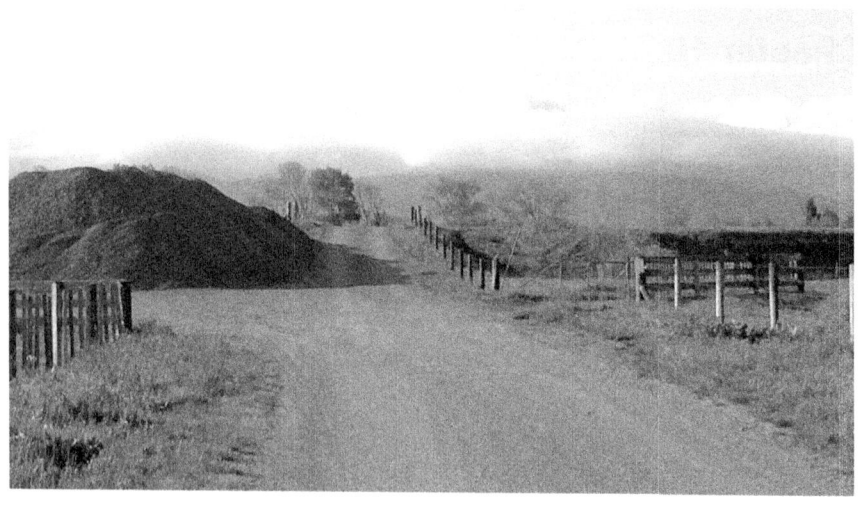

The stop bank or levee which protects us when the Manawatu River floods.

The right knee continued to be happy on the exercycle. The left knee was not quite ready to play along, but it wasn't far off. I began looking forward to when I could walk fast enough for Boots to comfortably walk with me.

On day 5 we cracked the exercycle with the left knee. It was a long time coming and gave me a real confidence boost. I pedalled backwards and frontwards. As the days progressed, I began timing the workout rather counting the number of revolutions.

I began doing 5 minutes in the morning after our walk but limited it to 2.5 minutes in the afternoon because, as usual, I tended to overdo things and then live with the regret. Now I could start to work on duration and increasing he exercycle's resistance, with the goal of eventually riding my real bicycle outside.

Week Fourteen

After the excitement of reaching new milestones in week thirteen, this week began with disappointment because the left knee decided not to co-operate on the exercycle for a couple of days. On day 4, I decided that mollycoddling the reluctant joint was not going to move us forward.

I opted for tough love and persisted through the pain barrier to do the forward rotation with the left knee. To hopefully avoid over-exertion, I limited cycling to 2-3 minutes, but did it three times a day after walking and knee-bending exercises.

My main discomfort was still during the first minute or so after getting up from sitting or reclining. A short period of walking around usually loosened everything up again. Fortunately, it was easy to regain comfort by putting my legs up, either on the couch or on a recliner chair.

Walking was going well. By carrying my poles on the outward journey, my normal walk was steadily improving. At the same time, using the poles enthusiastically on the way home helped maintain my upper body fitness to some extent. I still liked to use one pole when walking in town, because it alerted other people to my inability to move quickly.

Week Fifteen

For only the second time since my knee operation, it was too wet to go for a morning walk. I walked in the house, did knee-bending, then managed five minutes in relative comfort on the exercycle.

As usual, I got too keen on the exercycle, trying for several minutes three times a day. My lower back, which has had a relatively easy time of it for fourteen weeks, suddenly realized that biking muscles are more extensive than 'bending over' muscles. As a result, my whole body seized up. It felt wise to tone down the cycling activity to let the rest of the body adjust to the new type of exertion.

Now and then I had to remind myself that I was no longer fourteen and that an almost seventy-year-old body no longer has its old capacity to build muscle tone rapidly.

Longer walks of close to 2 km were feeling comfortable most mornings. I still walked out carrying the poles and used them on the return trip.

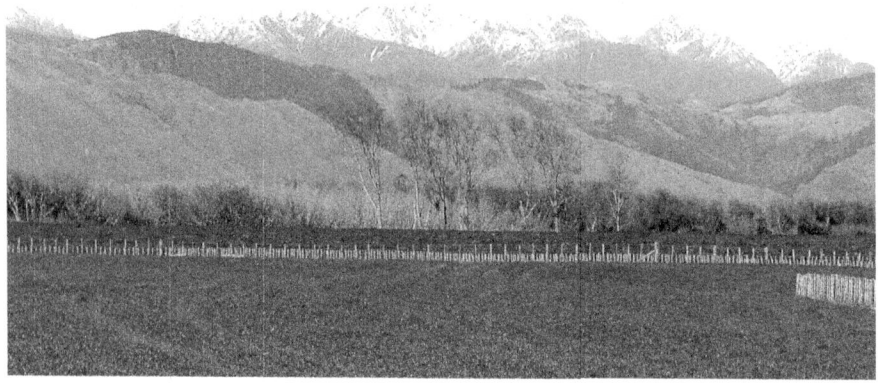

This sort of scenery during my walk always lifted the spirits.

Whenever I sat for an extended time, it still took some time to get back into movement. The greatest discomfort was during the first few steps.

Week Sixteen

The highlight of week sixteen was being able to put on my socks by bending one knee sideways resting on the other knee. I couldn't do it every time, but the beginning was there.

My lower back pain suggested that I should tone down the exercycle riding to two minutes morning and evening. I continued doing stretches twice a day.

Working at the computer was getting easier, but the knees still felt uncomfortably stiff on getting up every half hour.

Bending my legs sideways to put on my socks seemed to have activated a new set of muscles around the knees. They tightened up and for several days it felt like someone had applied a rubber hammer to each knee.

Week Seventeen

I increased my morning walk distance and on day 3 of this week I increased the exercycle time to 3 minutes twice a day without adding discomfort to my lower back.

On day 4, I noticed it was a bit easier to walk in the pugged muddy paddocks (while doing horse chores) without my stick.

Week Eighteen

This week I occasionally walked further than the end of the paved road toward the river. Walking on an uneven gravel track will help to stabilize the knee's side-to-side movement. I still carried my poles on the way out and used them on the way home.

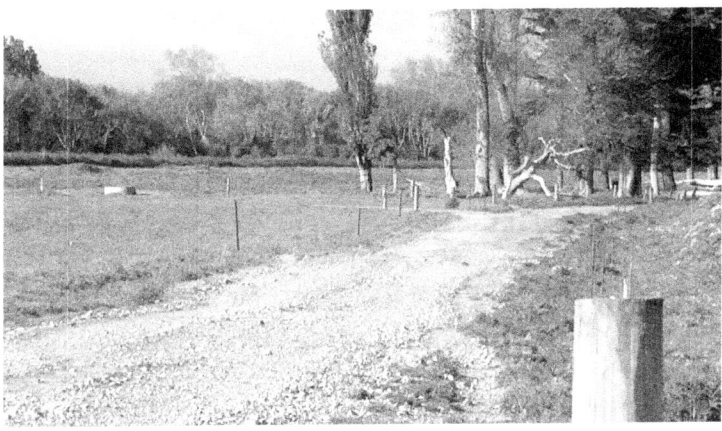

The gravel track that leads to the river.

Once home, I did knee-bending and then used the exercycle, gradually working up to five minutes at a time.

I was able to do more with my horse but suffered for it when I got carried away. I write and film a monthly horse training challenge for my Facebook page. Since the filming depended on good weather, it was easy to try to do too much during one session.

Week Nineteen

This week was much like last week. Some days were more comfortable than other days, probably in response to what I was doing. I could now work in relative comfort at the computer for three to four hours a day, taking my usual breaks to walk around every half hour. Evidently getting up and stretching every half hour is something that all people sitting at desks should do.

Sometimes I had generally sore legs when I woke up in the morning, but the knees were only uncomfortable when I was in motion. On my long morning walks, it took about half a kilometre before they really loosened up.

I was back to driving the car and it felt comfortable enough, although I wouldn't want to drive for much longer than half an hour.

Week Twenty

On day 2, we enjoyed a family outing in one of our city's lovely parks. My plan was to leave the car a half-hour's walk from the park's café, then walk to the cafe enjoying the spring blossom. My knees could have a rest while we had a snack, before walking the half hour back to the car.

However, construction work in the park meant we had to leave the car near the café. That meant we walked an hour's round trip to view the sights and return to the café.

I managed well with my Nordic Poles at the time. However, it took several days for my lower back to recover.

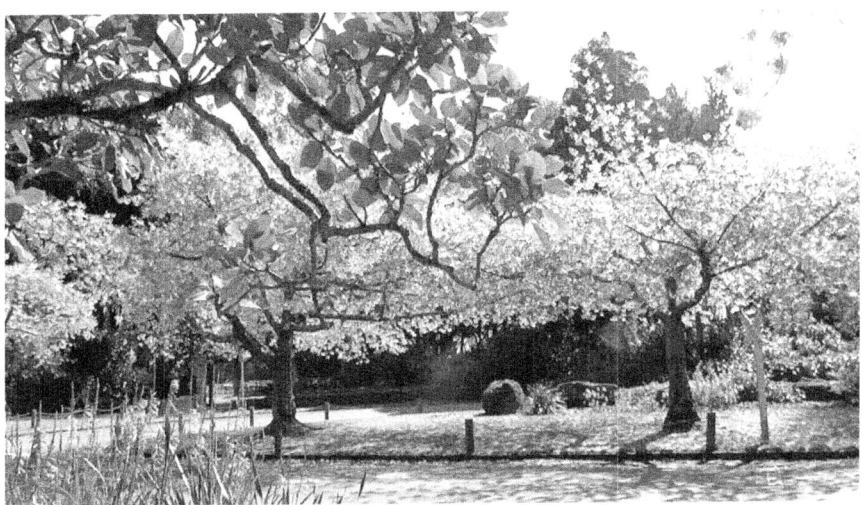

Cherry blossom at the park. This was my first major outing.

I think my body was (and still is at the time of writing) in the process of realigning itself with the different angles set by the new knees. Since the lower back muscles function to adjust the torso's position, it makes sense that they showed most of the strain. I also forgot to wear my usual walking shoes to the park, which probably made a difference.

I was sleeping well lying on either side and had not taken pain medication for many weeks. Most days I had the energy to do ground work with my horse, and I was gradually able to do more of the afternoon horse chores.

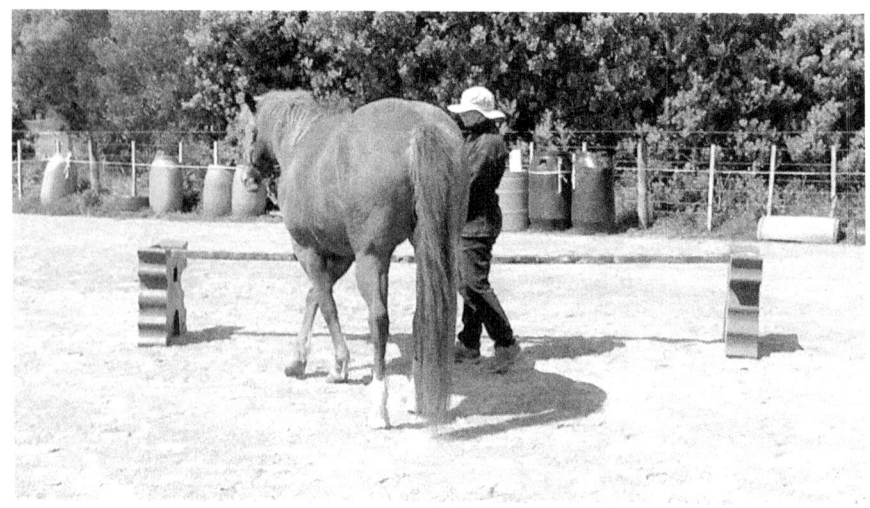

Working with my horse was my best therapy.

For shopping, I no longer felt the need to take a walking stick. If I had to go to the busy city center, I would take a stick because it let people know that I was a slow mover, which was especially helpful crossing a busy road.

Summary for Weeks Thirteen to Twenty

- Outward walk carrying poles horizontally, homeward walk using poles.
- Reached a walking milestone, the levee along the river, roundtrip distance about two kilometres.
- Right knee doing full forward revolutions on the exercycle.
- (Week 13) full backward rotation with the left knee and soon after, full forward rotation as well.
- Lifted one leg to rest sideways on the opposite knee to put on socks.
- (Week 18) Began adding short distances walking on the gravel track to the river.
- (Week 19) Drove car for the first time.
- Full hour of walking during an outing, body not happy the next two days.

Chapter Eleven: Weeks Twenty-one to Twenty-four

Week Twenty-One

My lower back was feeling stronger. Occasionally when I first got up in the morning, my right knee felt almost 'normal'.

It was easier to stride out on my morning walk, both without and with the poles. I still carried the poles first then used them on the way home.

Exercycle time was up to five minutes morning and afternoon and I gradually increased the resistance.

An attempt at riding my real bike failed miserably. The initial pressure required to start pedalling needed a lot more leg power than I had developed so far. The distance between seat and pedals also seemed shorter than on the exercycle and therefore required more knee bend.

I had to put my bike back into the shed. At some point I will gradually lower the exercycle seat, so it requires more bend, as well as continue to increase the resistance level.

My major discomfort was still right after getting up from reclining, working at the computer or traveling in the car. I thought that perhaps the knees were a bit quicker to 'rev up' again, but maybe that was wishful thinking.

We were getting close to the six-month mark. It was now clear to me that recovery is definitely a whole-year thing, just as the scary nurse told me before the operations.

On day 3 of this week, I extended my walking further toward the river along the gravel track. It brings the total roundtrip distance to about 3 km. Next goal will be to reach the river or walk further on the track.

Week Twenty-Two

This week I increased the resistance of my exercycle to level 3 and my leg muscles instantly complained about the difference. I compromised by cutting down the cycling time from five minutes to two minutes and will gradually build the time up again. It continued to feel as if I was always dealing with two steps forward and one step back to let other body parts catch up.

Walking is going well. My set base distance is about 2 kilometres, with occasional longer outings. I usually spent another hour at mid-day doing activities with my horse. Any knee soreness that arose with action dissipated once I put my feet up for a while.

Week Twenty-Three

The highlight this week was a full-day horse training clinic. I was pleased with how my knees coped with the long hours of standing and walking as well as the longish drive there and back. I took a chair with me and the other course participants were most helpful carrying it around for me from place to place.

I had taken over most of the driving to town for shopping and visiting. I put the exercycle resistance up to 4, after several days at 3. The knees had a strong reaction to that, but we (the knees and I) will persevere through the extra discomfort.

Week Twenty-Four

On the second day of this week a light frost and a crystal-clear morning with no wind begged for a longer walk. I'd been stopped from walking further toward the river by the stream of 700 dairy cows walking from their milking shed to their grazing venue at the time I usually reached the river levee.

To my delight, this morning it looked like the cows had passed by early. I could see them off in the distance and it looked like the gate had been shut behind them. Off I strode along the gravel track, grateful that the cow traffic had evened out the surface in places. I turned left though a gate to the river. It was my first visit to that quiet spot in over a year.

Heading back, I thought I saw the outline of more cows bobbing across the top of the stop bank half a kilometer away. "Oops," I thought, "There was another batch of cows coming". The cows' only option was to file along the narrow gravel track with electric fencing on either side. The gate open to their day's grazing was set at an angle, so I hadn't seen it from the road.

First, I thought I might beat them to where I turn off, but I soon realized that they were too far along for that. My best choice was to duck under the wire and make my way across very roughly pugged paddock closer to the stop bank. The cows and tractors had been though the paddock when it was wet, leaving the ground churned up and now sunbaked into a rough, hard, uneven surface.

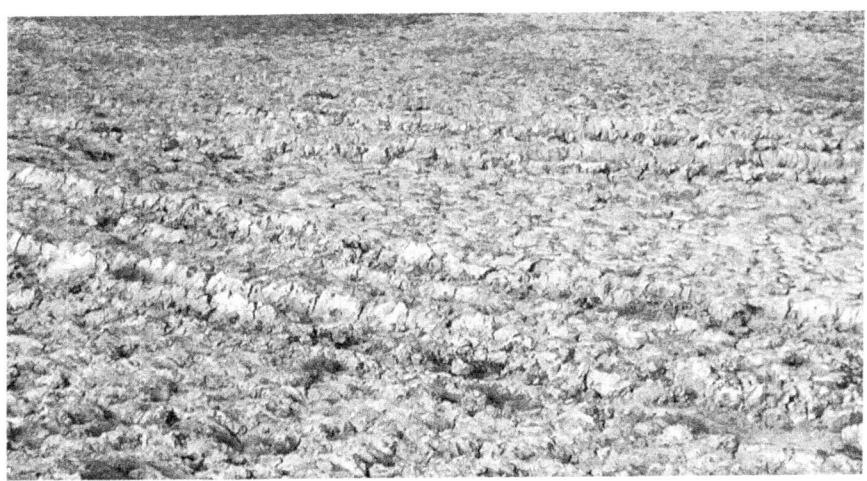

This was the pugged and sundried surface I was forced to negotiate. It took my knees several days to get over the trauma of having to slowly and carefully pick out each spot for my next step.

I found a set of tractor tire marks that resembled a railway line. Moving very slowly with my poles for support, I traversed the ruts. The last cows through the milking shed are usually youngest and most timid. A couple of groups stopped and stared at this unaccustomed person in an unaccustomed place. I knew enough animal behavior to widen the space between us. When this wasn't enough, I stopped and turned my back to them.

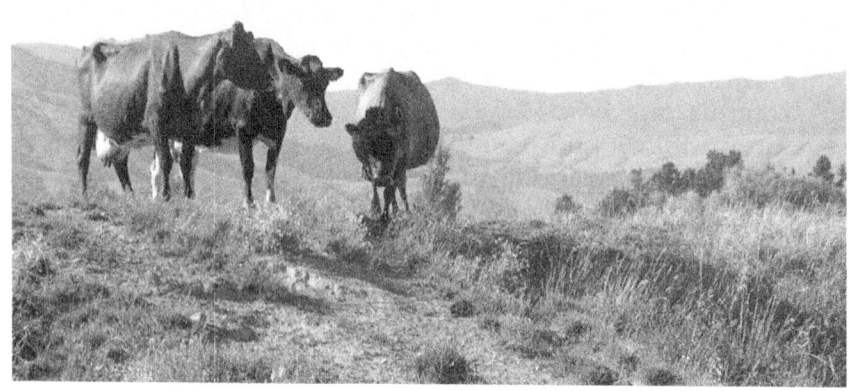

Some of the concerned cows.

My stopping and turning away gave the first group of cows the confidence to walk on down the track, but the very last group was startled into extreme immobility. It seemed that moving even further away was the only option if I didn't want to spook them. I inched my way over the pocked ground at an angle veering away from the cows and finally they sighed with relief and walked on.

I also sighed with relief and was grateful to finally reach the exit to the road. When I got home, my knees were clicking like I had never heard before. Next time I'll make sure the cows are grazing elsewhere. Bryan was beginning to wonder what had happened to me, since I'm usually back in half an hour. Today's 'activity' with Boots was sitting in a chair in her paddock with my sketchbook.

Summary for Weeks Twenty-one to Twenty-four

- Right knee felt noticeably stronger.
- Strove for two sessions of five minutes on the exercycle.
- Extended my walking distance on some days.
- Increasing the resistance on the exercycle put the knees and lower back into a sulk.
- Spent first whole day outdoors at a horse clinic.
- More driving felt fine.
- Extensive, unexpected walking on a rough surface caused a muscular backlash that lasted a few days.

Conclusion

This is probably an ideal place to finish this book. I feel confident that as long as I keep up my daily walking, knee-bending and exercycle activities, the muscles around my knees will continue to strengthen.

In a year's time I hope to update this book to add any highlights that may occur in the next six months.

NOTES:

Acknowledgements

This whole experience was made more bearable by the support of my husband who took over all my horse chores and has unfailingly boosted my spirits whenever they flagged. For a while he took over all the shopping and never failed to return with the chocolate bar I had included on the shopping list.

During the coldest part of winter, he lit the fire in our main living area first thing in the morning, so that I could emerge from my bed into a cosy space after enjoying the cup of herbal tea he brought to me in bed.

During the time I found it too agonizing to go for car trips, the extended family came to visit regularly. Thank you to Zoë, who cleaned Boots' feet every weekend until I was able to do it again. One tiny granddaughter, when she fell and bruised her knee, asked whether she now had to have new knees too.

Thank you to Bonnie Boon in Canada, whose editing skills have made this book much better to read. I enjoy your descriptions of prairie winters and summers from the comfort of the South Seas.

All the good wishes from, and on-going activities of, Facebook friends helped to while away the first couple of months when everything seemed too hard.

NOTES:

Appendix: Exercises I Found Especially Helpful

Note: After I stopped taking Codeine and Arcoxia in week four, I never took painkillers prior to exercise. I took Paracetamol very occasionally to help me sleep.

By not taking painkillers, I got an honest monitoring of how my body was coping with the rehabilitation of the muscles around my knees, as well as the new alignment of my whole body.

People vary in their pain tolerance, so setting up my own exercise schedule allowed me to rehabilitate at a rate that I could sustain over the long term. As the six-month mark came around, I knew that it would take considerably more time before my knees felt truly comfortable.

Early in the recovery it is tempting to avoid an exercise session because it is just so painful. I found having 'knee-bend' spots in various places around the house made it more likely that as I passed those spots, I would pause to do a few knee-bends.

Having set times to carry out the major parts of my 'rehab plan' was helpful. I also got a mental boost every time I could revise my plan to include new things I hadn't been able to do before.

Physiotherapists suggest that three or four exercise sessions (especially knee-bending) a day are more beneficial than two. A lot of published exercises suggest a certain number of repetitions. I opted to do repeats until I reached a certain level of discomfort, rather than follow a number. I subscribed to doing a little bit often, rather than a lot at one time.

My main thought is: Be patient with yourself. If you do too much, give your body time to settle down again. But every day, walk and do as much bending of the knees as you can manage. Doing less on some days is better than not doing anything. Don't give up.

Exercises

1. Lying or reclining, legs out straight, bend ankle to bring toes toward your face, then away. Try for 20 repetitions.

2. Lying or reclining, legs straight, push thigh muscles against the bed surface. Your heels will come off the bed surface slightly. Hold briefly then relax. Work up to 20 repeats.

3. Lying or reclining, legs straight, contract your buttock muscles; hold for a few seconds, relax and repeat. Work up to 20 repeats.

4. Sitting so your legs hang down, bring your leg up to straighten it and gently lower it again. Work up to 20 repeats.

5. Sitting on the edge of a chair, put your foot on a plastic bag (or have a woolly sock on a smooth floor or surface) and pull the foot as far back under the chair as possible. Use a ruler set in place, or masking tape, to visually mark how far back you can get your big toe. Achieving each new mark or measurement is great for feedback and motivation.

6. Lying down, lift each leg up straight from the hip, then flex the knee.

7. Lying down, starting with legs straight, bend each knee to bring its heel toward your butt, as far as possible without break-out pain. You can use a belt or rolled-up cloth to help pull the knee toward you. Having two new knees, I usually pulled them both back at the same time.

8. Increase walking distances, first with crutches, then with walking stick or Nordic Walking poles, then without help of poles or stick.

9. Take up Nordic Walking or Urban Poling if you possibly can. More physiotherapists are latching on the usefulness of this exercise to get people mobile and keep them that way.

10. Step over rails on the ground and lift the second leg up onto the rail. You might find places to do this in parks or use a curb or set up a couple of planks or a piece of 4x4. I happened to have rails I used with my horse. I found this one of the most useful exercises for the first few months of the recovery process. I usually did 12-20 repeats.

11. Knee-bending by stepping one leg up onto a surface and adjusting upper body weight to bend the knee as far as possible without break-out pain; hold for five seconds each time. Support with crutches or sticks to avoid any risk of losing balance. Gradually lift the leg onto higher surfaces. This became my main knee-bending activity because I could do it in many places.

12. Massage the muscles around the knees. I did this twice daily with my hands and my small, three-pronged, hand-held vibrating gadget.

13. Steps. Stepping up is considerably easier than stepping down. Be careful and use sticks for support. You don't want to slip or twist anything.

14. Holding kitchen benchtop:

    - March on the spot.

    - Stretch each leg sideways.

    - Raise heels to put your weight onto your toes, keeping body straight.

    - Raise toes to put weight into your heels, keeping body straight.

    - Knee bends facing the benchtop.

    - Knee-bends with back to the benchtop.

    - 'Kick the butt' exercise – i.e. bend the knee back and up; keep body straight.

15. Using a hallway:

    - Walk sideways to the left and the right.

    - Walk backwards.

    - Lunging steps.

16. Sitting in a recliner:

    - Sit so the knees lie across the gap between recliner seat and footrest. This is a knee-straightening exercise. Relax in that position until it becomes too uncomfortable. This stretches the muscles at the back of the knees. Strength will return gradually after regular repeats. It will stay comfortable for longer and longer.

    - Draw knees up and hold for as long as comfortable.

    - An alternative if you don't have a recliner is to sit in one chair and put your feet up on another chair so there is an air space below your knees.

17. Sitting or lying in bed, draw knees up and hold for as long as comfortable.

18. Exercycle:

    - Have the seat as high as possible.

    - Once you can get both feet on the pedals, play with just moving them back and forth rather than try for a full rotation right away.

    - Work with backward rotations first, as these are easier.

    - If you had both knees done at the same time, each will recover to its own timetable. It is best to avoid forcing the less willing knee. It will catch up eventually.

    - Be patient. The time will come when you switch from counting number of rotations to timing how long you stay on the exercycle.

- Try to avoid break-through pain as much as you can. If you keep things relatively comfortable, you will have stronger motivation to keep up your exercise schedule. Extreme pain tends to make us back off and do less.

- Some physiotherapists warn against being too eager to use an exercycle too early in the recovery.

19. Walk, walk, walk, walk. Several times a day. Walk. If it is wet or too cold, walk around rooms and up and down hallways and stairs if you have them handy.

NOTES:

NOTES:

Reference List

BOOKS

Gatica, Katie. (2016). *What to Expect with a Total Knee Replacement: A Patient's Guide to Surgery, Rehab and Beyond.* Amazon Kindle Edition.

Hargrove, Todd. (2014). *The Science and Practice of Moving with More Skill and Less Pain.* Amazon Kindle Edition.

Marshall, Lori. (2016). *Total Knee Replacement: 12 Weeks to Success.* Amazon Kindle Edition.

Stiles, Michelle. (2012). *Fast Track Your Recovery from a Total Knee Replacement: How to Eliminate Pain and Pain Medicine the Quickest Way Possible.* Amazon Kindle Edition.

YOUTUBE

I've chosen a few clips that I found easy to understand and helpful. There are lots more. Most of the material discusses single knee replacements. If you have both done together, as I did, you need an extra dose of patience and obviously twice as long to do the exercises.

It's also interesting to read people's comments. The main thing I noticed from the comments was that there is a huge variation in the amount of pain experienced as well as the length of the healing process.

This is not surprising, as there are so many variables including age, gender, general health, fitness before surgery, skill of surgeon, pain-relief drugs used, post-surgery care, support from family and friends, perseverance of the individual to do the exercises needed for recovery, paired with caution about twisting, falling and doing too much.

Overview: Knee Replacement: Dr. Mary O'Connor Reviews the Recovery and Follow-up (Mayo Clinic)
https://www.youtube.com/watch?v=JAQW073ZUx8

Surgeon's view: What To Do At Home After Total Knee Replacement (Talking with Docs)
https://www.youtube.com/watch?v=NJ-JspTqrHE

Physiotherapist viewpoint: Knee Replacement Rehab: Top 5 Mistakes People Make (Physical Therapy Video)
https://www.youtube.com/watch?v=HxxzeZHIPzk

Comments from someone who had a replacement: Total Knee Replacement Recovery - Answers To Your Questions (WS Westwood)
https://www.youtube.com/watch?v=mBdEHpxnJak

Using pillows to help sleeping positions: Best Position To Sleep After A Total Knee Replacement (Total Therapy Solution – Physical Therapy)
https://www.youtube.com/watch?v=xtDjQps7qDg

Exercises well explained and fully counted out, so you can use this clip (23 minutes long) and follow along to do your exercises: Post-Operation Total Knee Replacement Exercises (St. Mary's Regional Medical Center)
https://www.youtube.com/watch?v=QxrskgqIFhg

Bending and straightening exercises with a chair: After Knee Replacement: Two CRITICAL exercises! (Physical Therapy Video)
https://www.youtube.com/watch?v=qnm7tuSZmI0&list=RD xtDjQps7qDg&index=5

Foot-sliding gadget if you want to be more high-tech than a plastic bag or a smooth floor wearing fluffy socks: Simple Way To Increase Knee Bend After Knee Replacement-Real Patient (Physical Therapy Video) https://www.youtube.com/watch?v=blP1PtnS0AA&index=11 &list=RDxtDjQps7qDg

If you found this book helpful, a review on Amazon would be much appreciated.

Hertha James

Tiakitahuna, New Zealand

November 2018

Printed in Great Britain
by Amazon